AYURVEDIC HEALING

PANCHAKARMA

The Ayurvedic Art and Science of Detoxification & Rejuvenation

Dr. Suhas Kshirsagar BAMS, MD
Dr. Manisha Kshirsagar BAMS
Manas Kshirsagar AD

LOTUS PRESS

DISCLAIMER:
The information in this publication is for educational purposes only and is not a substitute for medical advice, diagnosis or treatment. For more information pertaining to your personal needs please see a qualified health-care practitioner.

ISBN: 978-1-6086-9241-5
Library of Congress Number: 2020935740

First USA edition 2020

Published by:

LOTUS PRESS

Lotus Press
P.O. Box 325
Twin Lakes, WI 53181 USA
800-824-6396 (toll free order phone)
262-889-8561 (office phone)
262-889-2461 (office fax)
www.lotuspress.com (website)
lotuspress@lotuspress.com (email)

Printed In USA

Acknowledgement

We have wanted to write this book for a long time. But we wanted to make sure this complex information was presented in a way that was accessible to the general population. So many hearts and hands have helped us shape this book. We are truly blessed to be able to do a day job that feels like our collective *dharma*. A path that allows us to meet, interact and help so many clients, students and seekers of health.

We sincerely thank our patients who shared their experiences and have allowed us to apply the ancient teachings of Panchakarma in a new design, that has proven to be very effective. Our deepest gratitude goes out to all the past and modern-day sages who have embodied the timeless Vedic wisdom throughout the ages. We are forever grateful for those who have laid the solid foundation for a wellness movement with Ayurveda & Yoga at its heart.

His Holiness Maharishi Mahesh Yogi, the founder of the Transcendental Meditation, called Panchakarma as a Veda Intensive Program (VIP) which provided a deep spiritual experience. Maharishi gave us direct experience and understanding to the most fundamental nature of reality.

Our deepest gratitude goes to Dr. Deepak Chopra MD for his inspiration, vision and friendship. His decades of work have helped Ayurveda regain the respect that it truly deserves.

Dr. Sheila Patel MD who is the Chief Medical Officer at Chopra Global was so gracious to write the foreword for this book. As a researcher, clinician and an educator of "Perfect Health", she was able to highlight the importance of Panchakarma. We thank her for her friendship and the hard work to be a leader in the ever-changing field of Integrative Medicine.

Drs. Vasant Lad, David Frawley & John Douillard are beacons of light that continue to guide and illuminate many lives. We express our deep gratitude for their wholehearted endorsement and blessings.

Marci Schimoff has always inspired us, her energy, insights and her "happy for no reason" attitude is genuinely appreciated.

We are grateful to our publisher Santosh Krinsky and his staff at Lotus Press who supported the project from its inception.

A big thanks to Nina Rogers whose design work have made the book cover and layout very attractive and pleasing. She has worked with us on all our earlier books and is an integral part of our team.

We would like to express our heartfelt appreciation to our family members, our dear parents, brothers and sisters who taught us the valuable life lessons of hard work, patience, contentment, and flexibility.

None of this could be possible without our staff at Ayurvedic Healing Inc. for their hard work and compassionate attitude. Our office manager Christy Boitz for her ever positive energy and smiling hospitality. Our therapists who are kind, experienced and absolutely love what they do! Something which is clearly reflected in their work. We work closely with many organizations such as Mount Madonna Institute, Chopra Global, Maharishi International University, Serenity Spa and Soul Yoga, Sivananda Yoga and we sincerely thank each and every one of them for their tireless pursuit towards the expansion of Vedic Knowledge.

Last but not least, we thank each other for the spirit of family and a sense of deep understanding, not only to write this book but to continue to inspire each other to serve our students and patients alike.

Wishing you Health and Happiness,

Suhas, Manisha, Manas Kshirsagar

Table of Contents

Foreword

We have learned that the established US health care model is not sustainable. There is more spending on health care in the US than ever before, yet there are more adults and children who are sick. We are noticing an increase in physical illness, as evidenced by an increase in the incidence of chronic disease, as well as an increase in mental health issues including depression and anxiety. What are we doing wrong?

The traditional healing system of Ayurveda would inform us this: we have stopped treating the human experience as a system of mind, body and spirit; we have stopped looking for the root cause of disease and instead are treating symptoms; we have not encouraged people to be their own healers by activating the innate healing systems that we already have; we have relied too heavily on pharmaceuticals instead of using food as medicine; we have overused expensive procedures instead of focusing on lifestyle; and we have ignored the importance of connection to community, nature and something even bigger than all of that.

What we currently need in health care are practitioners who are able to translate and carry traditional wisdom into the modern world. There are too few of these champions that hold the ancient wisdom that served humanity for millennia and can also communicate this wisdom to us in an accessible way. Drs. Suhas, Manisha, and Manas Kshirsagar are some of them. I feel honored as a physician to have them as colleagues and mentors. I have known this family of healers for many years, working directly with them all, and know that they not only hold a tremendous amount of knowledge, but also have been helping people heal for decades as practicing clinicians.

In my own practice with patients, I have seen time and again the futility of treating disease when the system itself is not receptive to the treatments. This happens when the body's natural detox mechanisms are hindered by the toxic burden, and when their level of stress is not allowing treatments to be effective. When our natural detoxification systems are not functioning optimally and our lifestyles are not healthy, we cannot heal.

One of the many aspects of Ayurveda that I appreciate is the fact that the practices do not force the body to do anything, they simply support the body in doing what it knows how to do naturally. As part of a complete panchakarma program, the oils heal us by providing anti-inflammatory support and binding of toxins, the massage helps to support the tissues and calm the nervous system, the herbs provide potent phytochemicals, such as antioxidants, which are necessary to repair free radical damage; the foods and spices support the microbiome and digestion which are necessary for detoxification and health.

Above all else, by providing recommendations for the mind and spirit, in addition to the body, Ayurvedic panchakarma is the most effective form of detoxification that exists. I hear often from patients after they have done various forms of Ayurvedic cleansing and detox that they notice a reduction in inflammation, improved energy and digestion, weight balance, and clarity of mind. In supervising a modified form of Ayurvedic cleansing at the Chopra Center for almost a decade, I have witnessed firsthand the benefits of this holistic style of detox. As you will appreciate from this book, panchakarma and other traditional Ayurvedic medical practices were not simply isolated esoteric procedures, but part of a comprehensive healing philosophy that includes body, mind and spirit.

As many traditional healing systems teach, the procedures done by medical providers must be supported by a healthy lifestyle by the patient before, during, and after therapies. When this is done, optimum health can be achieved throughout our lifespan.

Many of the practices of panchakarma are now gaining scientific validation. Concepts such as improving digestion and gut health, eating clean natural foods, aligning with circadian rhythms, are all becoming well accepted factors in creating health in the scientific and medical communities. Things that are not visible to the naked eye, so called 'invisible' forces, are now being renamed with terms such as 'biofield' and 'electromagnetic channels'. Some of the concepts may still seem foreign to our Western ears, but will no doubt have scientific explanations someday as we expand our understanding of how the mind-body system actually works. At the Chopra Center, we embarked on a landmark study to look at a whole-systems approach to health. The research design was not to look at simply one procedure or intervention, but to look at the benefits of a holistic Ayurvedic immersion. The SBTI (Self-Directed Biological Transformation Initiative) study sought to demonstrate the benefits in physical, emotional, and spiritual wellbeing after participation in an Ayurvedic cleansing and rejuvenation program. What we found is that by combining various practices as described in this book, in only 5 days, we can affect multiple metabolites in the blood to reduce the risk of disease, improve mood, and open people up to an expanded reality of self, known as non-dual awareness. We also found that these benefits continue even after participation, and help people create health on a daily basis at home.

I do appreciate the advances of modern science and will continue to use these tools when needed, however I can no longer imagine practicing medicine without also using the tools of traditional healing systems such as Ayurveda. To ignore these valuable practices, in my opinion, is becoming close to negligent care. It behooves anyone who considers themselves a health practitioner or healer to learn about the benefits of Ayurveda, including the important practice of detoxification and purification. We must also begin insisting that the conventional medical community open up to the benefits of other healing systems and practices.

Western medicine and Ayurvedic medicine do not have to be mutually exclusive, and in fact can work very well together. I have recommended Ayurvedic detoxification to many patients over the years to find that afterwards, their medications or supplements are more effective. Over time, as they continue Ayurvedic lifestyle practices that are right for them, many are able to wean off or reduce medications and supplements as their mind-body system returns to balance.

Fortunately for all of us, the healing system of Ayurveda is alive and well and the Kshirsagar family are among those that are bringing the wisdom of Ayurveda into our current society.

In this book, we dive deeply into a concept that has altogether been ignored in Western medicine. The word 'detoxification' has developed many connotations and has led to many fads, which is why it is so important to have books such as this to explain the true nature of detoxification and guide us toward complete systems of detoxification. As explained in the pages of this book, the ancient Ayurvedic practice of Panchakarma is key to reversing and preventing many chronic illnesses, both mental and physical, which are plaguing our population.

In our current day-to-day life, we are exposed to more toxins than ever before. Many environmental pollutants are now linked to chronic diseases and are at the root cause of many inflammatory conditions. They disrupt our hormonal and digestive systems and contribute to the development of disease. In addition, we have internalized socio-economic messages that we should be working constantly and pushing ourselves to our limits. These are just a couple of the factors disrupting our health and wellbeing. This book is an excellent point of reference for everyone to be able to understand the basics of detoxification and purification and be well on their way to a healthy and happy lifestyle.

In our modern age of science, we need to dedicate more research toward documenting the physiological shifts that occur with traditional therapies so that they are accepted into modern medicine and even covered by insurance. We need to find ways to blend the two so that we can help patients heal in body, mind and spirit. We need to educate physicians and other practitioners about the benefits of traditional healing systems. These benefits that have been observed over thousands of years, no doubt, can be described in the language of science over time so they become accessible to all. Not only can we not afford to lose traditional knowledge, such as that in this book, we must find a way to integrate it into our current health care system. Our survival depends on it.

This book will serve as a reference guide for all practitioners to bridge the gap between modern medicine and Ayurvedic healing. It will help to change the landscape of symptom management and shift to true healthcare the way it was originally intended.

Dr. Sheila Patel MD
Medical Director, Chopra Global

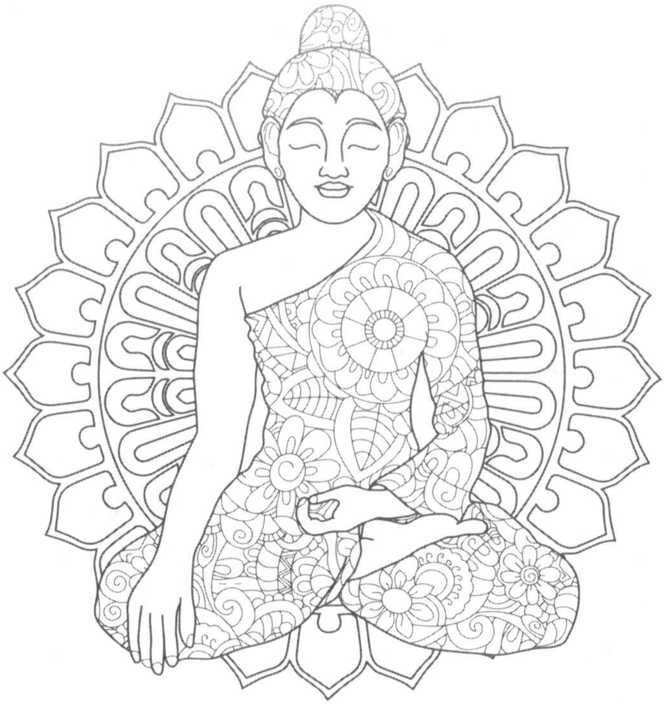

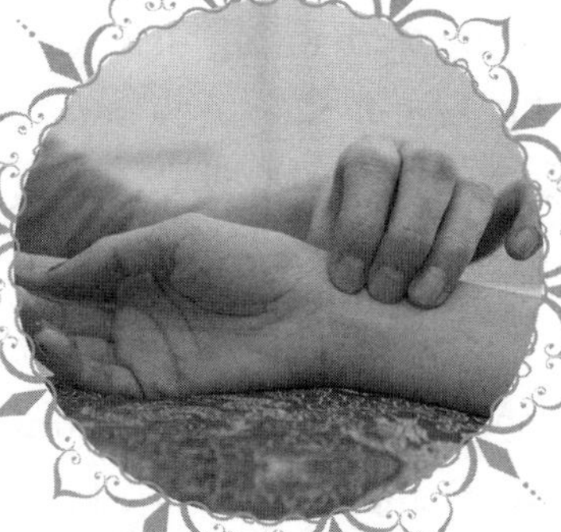

CHAPTER ONE

A DEEPER LEVEL OF DETOX

Like many of the people who call our clinic to ask about a panchakarma treatment, Jeanette had no idea how much her traditional lifestyle was affecting her health. She was a 56-year-old middle manager with a hectic but satisfying career. She traveled frequently for work and was often entertaining clients at restaurants. She worked long hours, even weekend hours, because she loved her job. Yet, she felt she was losing control of her health. She had been gaining weight slowly but steadily for about 15 years and felt she would need to lose more than 30 pounds to feel like herself again. But the weight wouldn't come off. She had hired a trainer to get into shape, then tried juice fasts and fad diets. Nothing worked. Many of our patients gain weight during the most demanding years of their careers. They try diets with more or less success and then give up. It's only when they have compounding health problems that they decide to make a drastic change.

In Jeanette's case, the trigger was joint pain in her wrists, shoulders and ankles. On some days it wasn't so bad, but on others she felt debilitated. More than that, she felt old, and that scared her. She went to the doctor for blood work and the results showed nothing wrong. Her doctor told her that she might have early symptoms of arthritis. This prognosis seemed like a dead end to her. No one wants to battle constant pain with over-the-counter medications. There is certainly no one who wants to do this for decades.

Of course, Jeanette is not alone. Many people work in careers that require long, late-night hours and travel. Lots of people eat frequently at restaurants or snack at unpredictable times and don't have a steady diet of healthy food. Some people have taken medications, such as antibiotics, for years to deal with an ongoing condition. Others have worked or lived in areas where there is a large load of chemicals in the water, air or soil. And some have turned to substances such as alcohol and tobacco to temper their levels of stress. Each of these presents a toxic burden to the body, one that can go unnoticed until symptoms present themselves and won't go away.

I felt Jeanette was an ideal candidate for panchakarma, the traditional Ayurvedic treatment to detoxify the body and balance its essential energies (or doshas). Although Jeanette didn't know anything about Ayurveda and told me that she was essentially skeptical of naturopathic healing, that didn't matter. She could benefit greatly from these treatments if she was willing to do the work to prepare for them. I gave her a preparatory diet that restricted her to eating healthier foods. She came to the clinic for seven days of treatment, during which her body was cleansed and rejuvenated. Afterward, her joint pain had evaporated and she'd also experienced several important insights about the direction of her life. She wanted to revitalize certain relationships and pursue some projects that she had been putting off. These are all normal outcomes of panchakarma treatment. Not only does the body recover its optimum level of functioning, but patients often report that they have more energy and enthusiasm for the things that are most important to them. Panchakarma has the power to cleanse the body and the spirit.

Many people come to Ayurveda because of a crisis like this. Traditional medicine has failed them and they need to reset the body's systems in order to regain good health. The first thing they need to do is to understand how toxins accumulate in the body to trigger pain or disease and how cleansing the system can help.

The Ayurvedic View of the Disease Process

Most people think of a detox as a superficial process. You change your diet, or take supplements, or abstain from harmful substances and the body does the rest. I am an advocate of all of these things. Unfortunately, many of my patients have health concerns that go beyond a poor diet. They need a multi-faceted approach to rid their bodies of excess toxins so that it can function optimally.

When you carry a burden of toxins from these various sources, you may gain weight, have low energy, achy joints, skin rashes, small things, nagging headaches that don't seem tied to any particular ailment. These are the tip of the iceberg in terms of your health. Eventually, they will tip over into actual health problems with your metabolism, heart or other major organ. Or you will be more likely to face injury from exercise.

People can walk around in this state of lower-level toxicity for years, reaching for cold medicines, headache remedies, allergy medications, antacids. They reach for all kinds of over-the-counter remedies when what they need is a deep tissue cleanse that will clear the body of all of this debris. We need to use a combination of heat, oils, massage and other treatments to get the body to purge the substances it has been holding on to.

According to the Vedic texts, the body is made up of different types of tissues, called dhatu. You will recognize some of them as they include the plasma and lymph system, the blood, the muscles and flesh, the fat, and the bones. So far, Ayurveda agrees with Western medicine in the types of tissues in the body. But Ayurveda adds an additional category, commonly called bone marrow. In Ayurvedic thinking the bone marrow includes everything encased in bone. So, in addition to the soft spongy tissues inside the long bones of our bodies, the bone marrow includes the brain (which is surrounded by the skull) and the spinal cord (which is encased in vertebrae).

In Ayurvedic thinking, these tissues have their own intelligence that runs the body's systems. Many of them are channels or fluids that pass through channels. The body is a constantly moving mass that has to take in nutrients, oxygen and fluids and use them or pass them along.

When we take in toxic substances, the body doesn't always know what to do with them. It may recognize these chemicals as foreign and pass them as waste, or it may encase them in fat where they can do limited harm. So, this means that your fat cells often contain the toxic substances that have entered your body through the air, through cosmetics, through pesticides in the foods, and through drinking water.

Although the body has valiantly fought to hide these chemicals and substances, they leak out. They accumulate and then they migrate to vulnerable tissues. Once the ama has settled into these tissues, it starts causing symptoms.

Interrupting the Body's Natural Defense Mechanisms

The body is designed to detoxify itself and it does so all day and all night. When you breathe, you are taking in nourishing oxygen and exhaling the gasses and molecules your body knows it doesn't need. When you eat, your body digests the nutrients and expels what it can't use. The skin sweats out toxins when you exercise or use a sauna. The blood is filtered through the kidneys and further cleansed through the immune system and lymph system. When you bleed, the body is using blood flow to push out impurities from the wound. The body has the internal intelligence to cleanse itself. So, why would anyone need further detox?

The answer is that sometimes toxins build up in the system and overwhelm the body's natural defenses. These can come from diet and lifestyle choices or from the environment. There are three types of toxins that can overtake the body's systems, they are:

ENDOGENOUS

Toxins: bacteria inside the gut that are especially prone to disease. A poor diet, high in saturated fats or processed foods and low on fiber feeds the bacteria in your microbiome that eventually become endotoxins. Poor lifestyle choices can increase the level of endotoxins in your gut and in your blood stream. This increases your body's level of inflammation which can lead to a host of chronic illnesses.

EXOGENOUS TOXINS

These are toxins found in the environment that can bring bacteria into the body. This toxic bacterium then sheds proteins inside the body that cause damage to healthy cells. Examples could be pollutants in the water, air and soil. They can also come from chemicals inside medicines or vitamin supplements or residual pesticides on our foods.

TRAUMA

Emotions also affect the body's natural function. Traumatic events at any time of life, but particularly in childhood, often leave a residue of dysfunction in the body's systems. A traumatic event or period of intense stress causes bodily inflammation that lasts months or years and can interfere with proper digestion, cardiac function and metabolism. Stress also gives a heaviness to the body and interferes with your natural desire to make good lifestyle choices. We often see patients who complain about fatigue, low energy, and mood swings, but their blood work is normal. Their doctors have no answers for them. But we know that this emotional ama can accumulate from childhood and contribute to the disease process.

Most people have a mixture of these toxins in their system. We accrue them from poor dietary choices and daily stressors. The type of toxin we are least prepared to battle is the exotoxins, the chemicals floating around in the environment around us. These chemicals accumulate in the body over time and get lodged deep in the tissues of the body. Once these compounds have been absorbed into the body's fat tissues, it stays there. The body's natural defenses can't pry it out.

The Most Common Environmental Toxins

You might think that you are only rarely exposed to dangerous chemicals, but the opposite is true. If you order take out in plastic containers, eat fruits and vegetables that are not grown in an organic environment, eat meat regularly or use detergents or cleansers in your home, you have been exposed to thousands of chemicals on a daily basis. When I explain to my patients that their health concerns may come from chemicals that have leached into their fatty tissues, they don't believe me. But the most common toxins are around us all day long.

PLASTICS

Nearly everything around us is composed of plastic. In fact, some of the clothes in your closet probably contain plastic or was spun from fibers made from recycled plastic bottles. The world produces 300 million tons of plastic each year and it's breaking down into micro particles that settle in the water and soil. Plastics also leech into our food when we store leftovers or takeout food in plastic containers. You make this worse when you heat food in a plastic container. If you wonder how this could be possible, just sit inside a new automobile and inhale deeply. That smell is the gasses exuded by the newly molded plastic and the various adhesives in the car. It takes many months for this smell to subside as the gasses dissipate, but they are still around you even if you can't smell them as clearly.

Scientists have long been studying the effects of plastic in the natural world. First, they looked at the tiny pieces of plastic worn down by the elements. These have been choking fish and birds for decades. But now those particles have become even smaller and rest in our water supply and the soil in which our crops grow. These microplastics contain chemicals that leech into our bodies when we drink them or eat plants grown near them. No one knows the effects of these microplastics when ingested, but they are not natural substances.

PESTICIDES

About 6 billion pounds of pesticides were used worldwide in 2012 and that number increases every year. Because so many weeds have become immune to older pesticides, the newer brands are even more toxic and contain more chemicals that can harm the human body. Many of these pesticides already reside in our bodies. A recent study tested for the presence of 212 chemicals in American subjects and found nearly all of them including trace amounts of 44 pesticides. When you ingest fruits and vegetables that were sprayed with these pesticides, your body stores them, and these chemicals can degrade your health. They may influence your chances of developing cancer or they can compromise your reproductive health.

MEAT PRODUCTS

Much has been written about the overuse of antibiotics in feeding livestock and how this contributes to super strains of bacteria that are resistant to common antibiotics. You may have seen meats labeled as "antibiotic free." While this is a good start, there are many other chemicals that meats are sprayed with or soaked in to make them safer to consume or easier to process. These include chlorine and ammonia to cleanse them of bacteria. Some meat and fish is sprayed with a gaseous compound including carbon monoxide to keep the surface color red for weeks and making it seem fresher than it is.

| COSMETICS AND CLEANERS |

Many of the substances we use to clean the house or our bodies also contain a host of chemicals that burden the body. There are more than 100 chemicals found in the home that are linked to allergies, birth defects, cancer and psychological disorders. Just a tiny fraction of the tens of thousands of chemical compounds created in the past 70 years have been tested to see if they are toxic to humans. There are more than 400 chemicals in cosmetics sold in the US that have been banned in other countries.

The problem is compounded with a poor diet and increased emotional trauma. In this case, the body accumulates its own sludge of food byproducts in the colon and intestines. The body can't fully release these without help.

What Panchakarma Does

Panchakarma is a full body detox on a cellular level. In Sanskrit, "pancha" means five and "karma" means action. So, a traditional panchakarma involves five essential actions that help remove toxins systematically from deep within the body. First, you go through preparatory treatments such as oil massage and a sauna. You will also ingest medicated oils. These pre-treatments, called Poorvakarma, dislodge toxins from your tissues and bring them into the main digestive tract. Then the five essential treatments push the toxins out of your system entirely.

There has been some research to show the benefits of panchakarma, but this research is by necessity limited. The treatments themselves are personalized to each patient. No two experiences are alike. So, it's difficult to do controlled studies on the effects of panchakarma. The one experiment that tried to measure these effects was carried out by the Chopra Center in 2016.[1] In this study, called the Self-Directed Biological Transformation Initiative (SBTI), participants were either placed in a relaxation control group or in the study group. The groups were similar in composition with regards to age, gender and body mass index. In addition, all participants had blood work done to look at lipid panels, blood sugar levels, among other things.

The control group were invited to enjoy their six day stay at the Chopra Center, with the condition that they not use the Ayurvedic spa services or have more than one alcoholic drink per day. They were cautioned against exercising more than they normally would on vacation. They were also encouraged to attend lectures on health and wellness.

The study group were prescribed several of the treatments that people normally go through when leading up to a full panchakarma treatment. They had daily massages, and saunas. They took prebiotic fiber and oils along with Ayurvedic herbs. They meditated and went to yoga classes. They also attended lectures on healthy eating and well being. After six days, the blood work was repeated in both groups and the findings were that key metabolites in the study group had shifted dramatically in just that short time. Their bodies showed less systemic

1. Peterson, CT, Lucas, J, John-Williams, LS. Identification of altered metabolomic profiles following a Panchakarma-based Ayurvedic intervention in healthy subjects: the self-directed biological transformation initiative (SBTI). Sci. Rep. 2016.

inflammation and better metabolism of cholesterol.

Even a partial preparatory treatment for panchakarma can have dramatic effects on the body. Full immersion into treatment has the power to reverse longstanding health concerns and restore you to optimum health.

It's important to understand that there are two types of toxins that affect the body. They are hydrophilic and lipophilic. Hydrophilic toxins get purged from the body through sweat and urine. Lipophilic toxins, by contrast, get encased in the body's adipose tissue. The body encases these toxins in fat cells because they can't be easily pushed from the body. These toxins have a molecular structure that is smooth and sticky, just like oil. They have an affinity for oil. Research shows that these lipophilic toxins are only removed from the body at a rate of 1 percent per year. This is the main difference between panchakarma treatments and other types of detox treatments. In panchakarma, the body is saturated with oils, massaged and then exposed to heat which draws the toxins out of the adipose tissue where they can be purged by the gastrointestinal tract.

CHAPTER TWO

WHAT IS PANCHAKARMA?

Ayurveda has been practiced in India for 4,000 years and panchakarma has always been part of that tradition. It was taught and studied in special colleges and practiced by individual physicians in every part of India. Over the years, monks who practiced visited other countries and took their learning with them. The most profound example of this migration came with the life and awakening of the Buddha. Siddhartha Gautama was born and raised in India but after his awakening to the suffering of the world, he left his home and family to travel in search of a solution to this suffering. He did not travel alone, but rather, in the company of an Ayurvedic physician, named Jeevaka. This legendary Ayurvedic physician gave out simple remedies and practiced healing on anyone they encountered. The Buddha considered that physical and spiritual ailments were intertwined and he wanted the monks who followed him and his teaching to be healers as well. These monks were trained in Ayurvedic healing and the practices of healthy living. In turn, they traveled throughout Asia and taught their own followers. This is how Ayurveda spread outside of India in the years following the Buddha's life. These monks also build academic centers and healing centers in many countries. These centers served in part as hospitals and nursing homes for thousands of years.

Until about 50 years ago, the panchakarma treatment was only offered in Ayurvedic centers in India. People considered this treatment to be a kind of pilgrimage of transformation that was much more significant and life changing than a series of medical treatments. This experience was reserved for people with chronic medical issues. It was seen as a place to turn when you had symptoms of type two diabetes, heart disease, unmanageable pain or any sort of deteriorating condition, either physical or emotional. If you had a health crisis that had been building for several years, you could go on a kind of retreat. You needed to leave your daily life and travel to an Ayurvedic center where you would live for two or three months under the supervision of Ayurvedic physicians and technicians. During your stay, you would eat the clean and simple diet served at the center. The people undertaking this treatment considered it a sacred experience in which every meal, every experience would contribute to healing your body and spirit. They might even shave their heads as a symbolic gesture that they were willing to live like a monk and to seek healing in the way that a monk seeks wisdom and enlightenment.

These Ayurvedic centers were usually built in spectacularly beautiful settings, either in a forest or near the ocean. Patients would live in this facility or in a village nearby. Patients could therefore take walks in nature every day and experience natural beauty as part of the experience. According to Vedic teachings, mother nature is a great healer in her own right. The plants and animals around us, the mountain vistas, even the ocean breezes contain healing energies that we can't see or measure, but they exist nonetheless.

You would eat simply and do exercises for the first month. The physicians would monitor your progress and start you on the poorvakarma, the preparatory procedures to loosen the ama in your system and get you ready for the actual treatments.

During the second month you would have treatments off and on. These would include deep massages, steam baths, herbal scrubs, enemas, emesis, or even leeches. Each treatment day consisted of yoga, simple stretches, walking, meditation or sometimes fasting. It was a daunting regimen, but effective.

During the third month, you would continue with a few treatments but mostly take rejuvenating herbs and continue with your exercise, meditation and healing to recover your strength and allow your digestive fire to rebuild. This is the phase in which you cement the habits you would have learned in the center about how to eat and how much. You would know your own body and how to properly exercise it. You might have gained a new love of meditation and nature and these things would help carry you back into your regular life. At the conclusion of your stay you would have completely rebuilt your health. You would emerge from the center and travel back to your family with a new vigor and a new perspective on the world.

In this old tradition, it was accepted that panchakarma must be done in a dedicated facility with trained physicians and that it must include all of the five actions and that it must take time. You can't be distracted by your ordinary concerns when you are trying to put your ailing body first.

In the past few decades, new Ayurvedic centers have opened up all over the world, and many of them provide a kind of panchakarma. It's a little bit different everywhere you go. In the US, for example, it is illegal to induce vomiting or draw blood, so those fundamental treatments are not available. The rest of the actions can provide great cleansing if done in the right combination and intensity.

Some Ayurvedic practitioners offer what they call panchakarma, but what is actually a few treatments give on the same day or for a couple of days in a row. Sometimes it involves only massage. Or there might be massage and steam baths. A few might add in enemas of various kinds. It's not easy to find centers with an appreciation of the classical tradition who can modify it for the patient's body type and schedule. In order to find the right treatment center, you have to understand what the traditional panchakarma entails and how it has been modified for the modern patient.

Pre-Treatment Preparation

Before a practitioner can embark on the five actions of panchakarma, he or she must take you through the process of loosening the ama, or toxins, that have been stored in the body's tissues. To do this, we use massage, steam heat, and lots of oil. These treatments are called poorvakarma. In Sanskrit, the word "poorva" means early, and the word "karma" means action. These include:

SNEHANA

The literal translation of this word means either oil or love. It can also refer to a bond, and this makes sense because when you ingest oil, it creates a coating inside the digestive tract, making everything smooth so that nothing else can stick to it. When you saturate the skin with oil, it bonds with the skin and permeates it, offering the nourishment the skin needs. With snehana, you will be swallowing oil and having it massaged into your skin to loosen the toxins both inside and out. Any herbs or medications added to these oils will sink into the skin and into the body.

| ABHYANGA |

This is vigorous massage with oils infused with herbs specific to your health needs. These oils permeate the skin. At the same time, the massage loosens the blockages that contain toxins in your body, allowing them to flow into the digestive tract where they can be eliminated.

| SWEDANA |

This word means to sweat or to soften, and that's what you'll do after the massage has finished. You might sit in a special steam bath that encases your body except for the head. Or you might have steam heat applied to areas of your body that are sore, such as the lower back or the joints. This opens the pores and allows the body to shed toxins.

| AMAPACHANA |

You will also be given some herbs to ingest to loosen up the ama in your body. This may come in the form of herbal teas. At our clinic we have several preparations that include powerful healing herbs including ginger and Trikatu.

The Five Actions

Once you have completed the pre-panchakarma treatments, the toxins in your body will have begun to flow out of the deep tissues and back into the digestive tract where the main actions of panchakarma can flush them from your system. In the classical tradition, there are five main actions of panchakarma. We don't perform all five of these in the United States because of regulations that restrict certain therapies. So, we have adapted the treatments in a way that you can reap the most benefits from these actions.

VAMANA

This is also known as therapeutic emesis, or induced vomiting. It's one of the treatments not performed in the United States. However, in India, this is a popular seasonal treatment. People go to outdoor camps in the spring and take herbal preparations that cause them to throw up. They don't experience any nausea, pain or distress. Rather, the herbal remedy helps to clear mucus from the sinuses, ears and eyes, and it opens the channels in the upper chest, neck and head.

VIRECHANA

For this, you take in substances that have a laxative effect on the body. This causes the colon and small intestines to empty. Not only are you clearing out any waste that has been trapped in the colon, you are also eliminating the mucus and toxins stirred up by the massage, oil and sweating during poorvakarma. It helps clear the liver, and the gall bladder. This has a powerful rejuvenating effect on the metabolism.

NASYA

Anyone who suffers from frequent colds or irritation of the nasal passages will benefit from Nasya, which involves administering drops of medicated oils into the nasal passages. This calms and clears those tissues and opens channels in the head and neck.

BASTI

This is another form of internal oleation. It brings medicated oils into the body through the colon. A practitioner will administer an enema containing medicated oils that coat the inside of the clean colon and then permeate the walls of the colon to repair it. These medical herbs also get absorbed inside the body. Remember that the colon helps to bring nutrients into the body. Any medicated herbs introduced here will be taken up and circulated throughout the system.

RAKTAMOKSHANA

This is another procedure not offered in the United States. In India, practitioners sometimes withdraw a little bit of blood from a patient to help calm and purify the blood. This can also be accomplished by placing leeches on the body. The leeches painlessly draw a small amount of blood and are then removed off the body.

You Must Prepare for Panchakarma

Many times, people call our center asking if they can book a panchakarma treatment right away. Maybe they have a friend or family member who has gone through the treatment and seen miraculous results. Maybe they have a doctor warning them about an imminent heart attack if they don't change their habits immediately. These patients are in a hurry, and yet the panchakarma demands time. You should never book such a treatment with any center who can take you right away without first meeting with you for a detailed history and without putting you on a preparatory regimen for at least a few weeks. The body has to be ready. It has to be ripened like a fruit. I say that you can't squeeze juice from a green mango. It just won't work. And if you try, you will bruise the fruit and damage the tissues. The same is true with the ama stuck inside your body. You need to loosen it up on your own for some weeks before it is ready to come out. You need to remove as much of the body's sludge as you can at home. Then you will receive more benefits from the concentrated treatments at the Ayurvedic center. Preparing your body reduces the discomfort you might otherwise feel in these treatments.

A few months ago, I saw a patient for the first time who was anxious to get his health back on track. A doctor had given him dire warnings about his cholesterol levels and insulin resistance. This man had failed to heed these warnings, but wanted instead a miracle cure from me. He'd read a little bit about panchakarma and thought the massage part sounded good. So did the steam baths. The enemas, he said, he could do without, but if that was a part of it, he'd go along. Whatever it took.

Unfortunately, the ama in his system was readily visible. He was carrying an extra 30 pounds and had a flushed and ruddy complexion. His skin was puffy and swollen. He had been eating restaurant food late at night for many years, including lots of fried foods and home brewed beer. The result was a longstanding battle with acid reflux and indigestion. He often stayed up late making music in his basement and rarely slept well. He also complained of near constant nasal congestion. At this point, his body was devoting all of its energy to expelling the ama that has backed up in his system. He needed to work to open the channels and show his body some much needed attention.

The body is trying to cleanse itself constantly. It does this with breath, urine, stool, sweat, and anything that emerges from coughing and sneezing. When you can't lose weight, can't digest food without pain, can't breathe because of congestion, and can't sleep, your body is giving you strong signals that it has been overwhelmed by contaminants. To put someone on a table and douse them with oil and deep massage would further traumatize the body. The first step is to change the diet and daily routine of the patient so that the body can work its own magic on the toxins. Only then will it be ready for more intensive measures.

I told him that it would not be possible for him to have any panchakarma treatments until he had demonstrated some changes. First, he had to completely give up alcohol for the next 30 days. This was going to be hard for him because he prided himself on brewing his own beer and giving it out to friends. It was his favorite hobby, and made him very popular. But he said he would try. Second, he had to give up restaurant food for the month. I told him to eat an early meal at home, go make music for a little while, but be in bed by 10:30 every night. He had to cut back on meats and eat many more vegetables. No coffee in the morning. He would be drinking green tea instead.

He seemed dubious, but I told him to try it. What did he have to lose? I knew that any changes he made would reap benefits tenfold on his beleaguered body.

A month later, he came back and told me that he'd lost 11 pounds. That alone seemed like a miracle to him. What's more, he had gone to the doctor and his blood work showed a real improvement in his fasting glucose. And his cholesterol had dropped by 30 points. Even his doctor was astonished, saying that he'd never seen that dramatic an improvement in such a short time. The doctor said to him, "Whatever you are doing, keep doing it."

It was a remarkable transformation. He had new energy, new creativity and he felt great. Yet, he was still not ready for panchakarma. The skin still seemed a little swollen and his pulse betrayed a continuing pitta aggravation. Surely, his body was rejoicing at being able to shed some of the sludge in his colon, and being able to digest food properly. His acid reflux had disappeared and his sinuses had mostly cleared. But there was more for him to do. The panchakarma is for cleansing of the deep tissues. He was still working on the surface level. His body had many more joys of good health to experience with his new diet. And I wanted him to begin to exercise in earnest, gently at first and then with more rigor. In time, perhaps in a few months, his body would be ready for a more comprehensive cleanse.

This is the type of consultation you should expect from any pre-panchakarma treatment. You want to get the right advice at the right time and you want to work with an Ayurvedic therapist who understands that you can only get the most out of this special treatment with the right preparation. You will need to be able to adhere to a special diet for three to four weeks and you will have to do some cleansing treatments at home to clear out your bowels. Even those patients who come to me and have had excellent health regimens for many years need to do some preparation. Specifically, they need to take in prescribed amounts of oil every day for about three to seven days before they start. Everyone needs internal lubrication to prepare the digestive tract for the treatments themselves.

If you don't take these steps, the treatments become more difficult to endure. I've seen people who have had panchakarma at other centers where they weren't properly prepared and they suffered from headaches, rashes, cramps and other ailments during the treatments and for weeks afterward. I tell people to think of panchakarma as a sort of dream vacation for your health. Think of it as a once-in-a-lifetime experience for your body. You want your body to be fully prepared so that it can enjoy every moment.

Giving Up Distractions

Some people believe that a panchakarma is like a spa treatment, in that they will come to the center, get their treatments in the morning, and spend the rest of the day doing work or managing their lives from afar. This is not the case. Because of the intense nature of the experience, you will need to plan to devote all of your time to gentle activities that support each day of treatment. This will mean a prescribed diet that will be light and clean. It will mean taking time away from the details of your regular life.

This means putting away the cell phone for the duration of the stay. You will not be working, scheduling meetings or checking in at work to make sure they can survive without you. You will not be watching television, listening to podcasts or zoning out to YouTube. Your body, mind and spirit need to stay focused on your one goal of improving your health. This electronic fast is mandatory. Remember that you are entering a space that will be a complete counterpoint to modern life. You will be leaving behind the notions of running around, juggling details and taking care of others. Instead, everything will be focused on taking care of you. Some people find this incredibly relaxing, while others have so completely forgotten how to receive attention and care that they feel disoriented at first.

In the classical tradition, you were expected to come to the retreat center and live there for two to three months and engage in treatments as your physician saw fit. In the modern era, we often schedule the treatments by the number of days you have to spare. You might come for three days or five days or seven days. And so, there will be several procedures you go through on each day. These will be tailored to your body type, the type of toxic aggravation your body shows in a pre-treatment physical. These will also be adjusted day to day based on your physical or emotional response to each procedure. In addition, you may be asked to journal or meet with an Ayurvedic physician each day who will ask how you are faring and check in on how your body is responding.

I remember one woman coming in for panchakarma who could spare just three days. She had been a successful life coach who had become an even more successful motivational speaker. She traveled extensively and was constantly in meetings and on the phone all day. She had a pitta constitution that perfectly suited her job. She had a dazzlingly confident presence and I had no doubt that she had changed many lives with her talks.

Yet, she was plagued with insomnia and had difficulty controlling her anger and perfectionism. More than that, she felt lost and stuck in her life. And she was having headaches and was beset by seasonal illnesses that left her bedridden for weeks at a time.

Three days is not a lot of time in which to work. Still, we tailored a regimen for her that would address these health concerns, and in addition, I told her that she needed to spend the three days with us in complete silence. She was surprised, but agreed to surrender her cell phone and to speak not one word for three days. She stayed at a monastic center nearby where they also expected silence. During the treatments, her technicians knew not to ask her any questions and during our daily meetings, I would merely take her pulse. If she needed anything, she could write a note on a piece of paper.

At the end of her stay, once she was allowed to speak again, she told me that she felt unstuck for the first time in years. She felt lighter and healthier, but more than that, she had decided to make some sweeping changes in the way she structured her life and her business. Further, she thought about why her marriage wasn't working and had some ideas about how she had contributed to these problems. She could see that the way she was treating others wasn't working for her.

The Power of Silence

There are many meditation retreats that use silence as a way of enhancing spiritual progress. The Chopra Center hosts one of these events, called the Silent Awakening, which is a 7-day event for people who wish to spend an extended time without speaking as they pursue their meditative goals. It sells out each year as more than 200 people come to the center and spend the entire week engaging in yoga classes, meals and meditation sessions without speaking. It can seem eerie to see so many people walking around and not chattering to each other, but it is also very beautiful. The watch the sunsets together. They eat together. They are definitely communing, just not speaking. Once a day, they write down questions and Deepak Chopra takes the stage to answer them. I've seen people looking a little lost because they don't know how to encounter others without the cover of mindless chatter. A few people cry a little bit as they deal with feelings they've pushed away. But everyone emerges from this retreat with a new sense of purpose and a new sense of themselves.

It's a little bit unusual to ask people to remain silent during their panchakarma treatments, and yet it can be surprisingly effective for the right person. Some people are so busy, and have so much chatter in their heads that they can't think straight. They can't experience their moment to moment lives. And that means they can't commune properly with the body. When someone like this is plunged into silence, they can't use speech to mold the world around them and to bend others to their will. At first they feel helpless, but gradually they become vulnerable and open to new ideas. They become aware of old thoughts and previous hurts they have been pushing away. It's very purifying to put away words for a period of time and let the body and the subconscious do the talking. This silence coupled with journaling can bring startling insights.

When silence is used as part of panchakarma, it is even more transformational. We are working on the body to massage away these old blockages. This allows toxins to flow more freely out of the tissues. Then we use enemas or steam to pull it out through the skin or the colon. The oil massages and pastes further open the body's channels. With sensory therapy, we clean out the sinuses and provide a sensation of complete relaxation. The silence merely enhances all of these things. Gradually, you begin to feel the transformation in your body without having to describe it to yourself or anyone else. Now, you can put your body and your health at the center of your reality, where it belongs. Once you've done this inside the treatment room, you can do it again when you leave. This ability is life-changing.

The Rejuvenation Phase

At the end of your treatments, you will be going back into your regular world. Instead of being away for two to three months, as in the classical tradition, you will have been away for just a few days—or perhaps a week. You will have gone through many experiences, felt many new sensations, changed your diet and changed your health outlook. You will go back into your life altered and may be wondering how to acclimate back into that world.

A good center will prepare you for your return to daily life. During your panchakarma treatments, you will be given a modified diet that allows you to take in nutrition without overwhelming your body. The usual Western diet is so high in unhealthy fats, sugar and salt and do low on nourishing vegetables and grains that it won't be appropriate for you at this time. Instead, you will be eating small meals that might include kichadi, a traditional soup made from rice, mung beans, healing spices and ghee. Or you might be eating simply rice or a rice porridge. You won't be very hungry during your treatments, but you should be taking in some food during the day. There may be some portions of your treatment regimen that will include fasting.

As you finish your treatments, your practitioner should be talking to you about the daily routine and diet you will need to stick to in order to make a smooth transition to regular life. You will probably start at home with a highly modified diet of kichadi soup. You will abstain from meat, alcohol and coffee at first, along with most vegetables. As the days continue, you can include more vegetables in your regimen and finally, you will be able to return to a healthy diet of mostly vegetables and some small portions of meat. Many of the people who go through panchakarma want to keep eating in the light and healthy way they've learned to eat at the center because their bodies feel so good and they don't ever want to feel heavy and dull from eating junk food. Others try to go back to their old diets and find that their favorite foods and candies no longer taste good to them.

In addition to diet, you will want to engage in some exercise after your panchakarma, but again you don't want to overdo it. Let the body acclimate slowly to more exertion. Your practitioner will likely tell you to take prescribed herbs for a few days or weeks after your treatment to help facilitate recovery. Even though you may feel light and strong, you will want to take care of your body and not overdo it with eating and exercising right away.

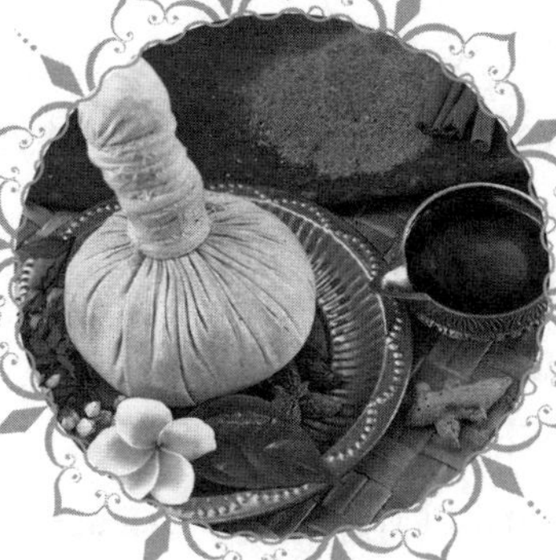

CHAPTER THREE

ARE YOU A CANDIDATE FOR PANCHAKARMA?

This intensive treatment addresses toxins that have lodged deep inside your tissues. You won't be able to see or feel these toxins and your regular doctor won't be able to point to them on a chart or scan. In allopathic medicine, it was long assumed that you can only treat the body once evidence of disease has been identified. After the body stops functioning properly, the doctor can make a diagnosis and select a treatment. It's only in more recent decades that western medicine has come to the conclusion that many diseases manifest in the body after a long period of distress. Metabolic disorders, heart disease and arthritis are some examples. It's only after decades of distress that the body succumbs to advanced chronic illness. According to Ayurveda, the body is always offering information about how it is operating. The body has its own innate intelligence and is always trying to find balance. By paying attention to the body's signals early on in the disease process, we can avoid chronic diseases.

Past injuries also contribute to toxic accumulation. If you suffered injuries in an accident or from playing sports decades ago, toxins can collect in and around these old injuries. We sometimes think that the affected body parts didn't heal completely and that this failure to heal is what causes nagging pains years later. Actually, these body parts may have been weakened and these spots can collect ama over the years. A panchakarma treatment helps drain out the accumulated ama and rebuild the tissues so that the body can function pain free.

Let's add to that the possibility of emotional distress. New studies show that children exposed to emotional trauma, neglect or abuse are many times more likely to experience disease, depression or addiction as adults. That's in part because the mind carries these old injuries, and because the body and mind are so closely linked, the ama collects throughout the body as well. I see patients carrying trauma from decades before that is still affecting their health. In the years after the trauma they told themselves to forget about it and move on, but the mind is wily about not letting things go completely. It stores these feelings of helplessness and fear. At some point, they awaken. One of my patients remembered her parents' divorce from when she was four years old. It was a harrowing time for her because she didn't know who would have custody and each parent was dating a lot of new people for several years. What she had really felt was abandonment and the sense that life was unpredictable and unfair, and that the people in charge of her life didn't care about her. She didn't really remember these feelings but they were stored up inside her. Then, at age 28, a longtime boyfriend broke up with her suddenly and her health spiraled out of control. She became depressed, and broke out in rashes and had terrible migraines. Her doctor couldn't figure out the cause. But I talked with her about her physical symptoms as well as her emotional history. She came to realize that some of the old emotional wounds were contributing to her physical symptoms. She realized that she needed more than medical treatment. She also needed to go into therapy after the panchakarma. Most times, just pointing out that physical and emotional ailments can be intertwined helps people understand their health in a broader sense.

Ayurvedic Stages of Disease

In order to understand whether you would benefit from a total body detox, you might want to know more about how disease manifests over time. We are often told that disease springs up suddenly. In reality, most people are accumulating toxins that can progress toward disease or injury. In Ayurveda, we understand that there are stages of disease that begin long before symptoms are likely to be felt or measured. What's great is that if you are aware of the early stages of the disease process, you can take preventative measures to reverse the process and maintain health through every stage of life. Only the final two stages of disease represent conditions that are likely irreversible.

ACCUMULATION

In this first stage, the ama is building in the system. This can be caused by a sedentary lifestyle and poor diet. You don't get the exercise that you know you should and maybe have habits of eating junk food or staying up late at night watching TV or doing online shopping when you know you should get more sleep. You might notice this accumulation phase as the normal malaise of a busy life. You have less energy than normal and maybe more prone to frustration when faced with small inconveniences. In terms of physical symptoms, you might notice that you've got some stomach issues or minor bowel issues. Things feel a little off, but the symptoms go away quickly. This accumulation can also start at a particular time of year. If you have a kapha body type, you'll notice that you are prone to sickness in the spring season. This is when accumulation starts for you if you aren't taking care of yourself. Pittas struggle in the heat of summer, while vatas are more prone to feeling scattered or depressed in winter. The symptoms at this stage tend to be seasonal and they also seem to be temporary, which is why they are so easy to ignore.

AGGRAVATION

Once the ama has accumulated enough in one location, it starts to make more persistent trouble. You have a cold that takes two weeks to clear up. You have a headache that's bothering you for several days in a row. You might have a little bit more trouble digesting your food. The stomach or bowels want to rebel a little bit when you eat foods you know you shouldn't. You might be putting on weight and telling yourself that you'll go on a diet soon, or get more exercise soon. You might have persistent congestion in the morning or other nagging symptoms. Emotionally, this is when people start to complain to their friends about being stressed out. The body is beginning to call out to you to please take better care of it. Most people ignore these pleas. In fact, there's a great temptation at this stage to reach for comfort foods and bad habits as a way to feel better, however temporary this feeling is. This is a great opportunity instead to clean up your diet, get on the right schedule for your body and perhaps take some cleansing herbs in tea in order to get lasting relief.

DISSEMINATION

This is when ama leaves the digestive tract and spreads to other parts of the body. This is what I call the medicine cabinet phase. When patients come to me, they are often at this stage of disease. They have a medicine cabinet full of remedies that don't actually help. They are taking pain relievers for persistent aches in the joints. They are taking decongestants for constant sniffles. They have headaches at the end of every day. Constipation makes them feel congested and lethargic. For every one of these ailments, they have a pill or liquid to help keep the symptom at bay. And this is the stage where weight gain seems intractable. No diet will touch those extra pounds. And no diet lasts because when your energy is low you can't follow a diet. The body has lost its compass. They come to me asking for powders and herbs but we are past that point now. The body at this stage needs a complete reset. It can come from panchakarma but it can also come from months of work to retrain your habits and get the body's energy flowing again.

LOCALIZATION

As the ama continues its spread, it will eventually find a vulnerable spot in which to land. This might be the site of an old injury, or it might be some tissue that has been compromised before by repeated illness or infection or surgery. Wherever the ama lands and takes hold, it begins to disrupt and damage the tissues in this area. This is the phase when many people consult a doctor and present with multiple problems that seem unrelated. They wonder what their constipation could have to do with their back spasms or their sudden acne. They wonder what their insomnia could have to do with their stomach ulcers or anxiety. But these things are related to the root cause of a body that is out of sync with itself. At this stage blood work may show some troubling signs. You may have slightly elevated blood pressure or higher blood sugar levels, but in most cases doctors won't be able to prescribe anything. This is the stage at which many people need something more drastic, such as panchakarma to reverse the course of disease.

MANIFESTATION

This is the stage at which traditional western medicine will intervene. Now you have repeating symptoms that no one can ignore. At this stage the ama has reached a global level in the body. There is enough systemic inflammation that you may have markers for metabolic disease or heart disease. There may be diminished liver function. And you have all of the symptoms that go along with this including low energy and libido, perhaps even depression. Regardless of how much you eat, your body will not be able to absorb nutrients to nourish the tissues and there's very little that can be done to reverse course.

DISRUPTION

This is the end point for ama. By this time, the body's energies are completely distorted. Physical symptoms may include noticeable inflammation, a foul smell to some tissues, or even chronic infection. At this point, the health problems are chronic and systemic.

Ayurvedic Treatments for Symptoms

The purpose of panchakarma is to halt this disease process at the earliest stages and reverse course. By reaching into the tissues to soften the ama and remove it, you can rebalance the body and open the natural channels of energy.

It might be helpful to understand the two theories of healing that often compete with each other. The first of these is called shamana, which means relief from symptoms. Whenever you reach for a pain reliever or over the counter decongestant, you are using this theory of healing. The idea is that relieving the symptoms is the same as curing the condition. It seems obvious. The symptom is the problem, so removing the symptom brings relief. A decongestant will open up the sinuses temporarily, but it also dries out the sinus tissues and the tissues throughout the body. Take this same decongestant over the course of several days and your body will dry out, which could lead to other problems. Ayurveda does use shamana in some cases. When health concerns are small, they can be handled fairly quickly. The problem is when you confuse the symptom with a larger undiagnosed problem.

In Ayurveda, we know that many health problems need a different approach, known as shodhana. This refers to diagnosing the course of the illness, the entire problem, in an effort to make it go away. For example, if you had congestion, your Ayurvedic practitioner might have you breathe in herbal steam. Then give you bitter drops in each nostril and ask you to inhale. This will produce ferocious sneezes. And you will be draining fluid for several hours. That probably doesn't sound very pleasant. But it's curing the problem of congestion rather than masking it with drying decongestants that draw the virus back into your tissues. Instead, the treatment triggers the body to drain out the fluid containing the irritant. You've gone through a few sneezes and a few hours of runny nose. But in the morning, you are clear on a physical and emotional level.

Panchakarma is a shodhana treatment. It is a total body commitment for several days in a row, but at the end, your body's channels will be clear and open.

Detox Quiz

Many patients are interested in these treatments because they have tried to follow healthy habits but are not seeing progress in their health and vitality. They still have some insomnia or other symptoms that are bothersome. One of the things we ask patients to do is to take a quiz about their level of ama, or toxins in the body. With this information, your practitioner can devise a plan for treatment that will be most effective for you.

In an appointment before the panchakarma, your practitioner will look at your tongue, take your pulse and get a sense of the actual level of toxic burden in your body. Even if you've led a fairly healthy lifestyle, you can still have a buildup of toxins from pesticides in the environment, industrial chemicals, mold in your home, plastics or other exogenous toxins that you've ingested without realizing it.

Answer each of these questions. You can circle your response. A level of 1 means that you rarely experience this. If you circle 4, you are saying that you experience this often or severely. Leave the question blank if you've never experienced this symptom.

	QUESTION	ANSWER
1.	I experience belching, gas or heartburn after eating.	1 2 3 4
2.	Certain foods cause stomach upset or indigestion.	1 2 3 4
3.	I feel bloated and uncomfortable after I eat.	1 2 3 4
4.	I sometimes go a whole day without producing a bowel movement.	1 2 3 4

	QUESTION	ANSWER
5.	My stools are loose and unformed.	1 2 3 4
6.	I have constipation.	1 2 3 4
7.	I crave carbs and sweets.	1 2 3 4
8.	I retain water.	1 2 3 4
9.	I have been trying to lose the same excess weight for many years.	1 2 3 4
10.	I become easily intoxicated after one or two drinks.	1 2 3 4
11.	My pulse speeds up after I eat.	1 2 3 4
12.	I'm sensitive to chemicals, such as perfume, cleaning solvents and tobacco smoke.	1 2 3 4
13.	I have fatigue or joint pain.	1 2 3 4
14.	My sweat has a strong odor.	1 2 3 4
15.	My urine has an unusually strong odor.	1 2 3 4
16.	I experience pain in the lower back.	1 2 3 4
17.	I urinate frequently.	1 2 3 4
18.	I have asthma.	1 2 3 4
19.	I experience shortness of breath, or chest congestion.	1 2 3 4
20.	I sometimes experience a rapid heartbeat when I have not been exercising.	1 2 3 4
21.	I flush or blush for no reason.	1 2 3 4

	QUESTION	ANSWER
22.	I sometimes wheeze or have trouble breathing.	1 2 3 4
23.	I experience recurring cold sores or fever blisters.	1 2 3 4
24.	I have acne that flares up without warning.	1 2 3 4
25.	My skin is sensitive to chafing.	1 2 3 4
26.	I have psoriasis.	1 2 3 4
27.	My fingernails are grooved or split easily.	1 2 3 4
28.	I have puffy eyelids or bags under my eyes.	1 2 3 4
29.	My eyes water or are itchy.	1 2 3 4
30.	I have dark circles under my eyes.	1 2 3 4
31.	The whites of my eyes are yellowish or bloodshot.	1 2 3 4
32.	I have excessive discharge in my ears that is hard to clear.	1 2 3 4
33.	My ears sometimes become infected.	1 2 3 4
34.	There is a ringing in my ears.	1 2 3 4
35.	I experience congestion even when I don't have a cold.	1 2 3 4
36.	I have seasonal allergies, or they have grown worse lately.	1 2 3 4
37.	My nose runs even when I don't have a cold.	1 2 3 4
38.	I have a yellowish or white coating on my tongue.	1 2 3 4

	QUESTION	ANSWER
39.	I experience mouth sores or canker sores.	1 2 3 4
40.	My mouth, nose or eyes are frequently dry.	1 2 3 4
41.	I have difficulty swallowing or gag easily.	1 2 3 4
42.	I have headaches.	1 2 3 4
43.	I sometimes experience dizziness or lightheadedness.	1 2 3 4
44.	I have pain or swelling in my joints.	1 2 3 4
45.	My knees or hips ache or I have backaches after exercise.	1 2 3 4
46.	I have aches and pains every morning.	1 2 3 4
47.	I'm easily fatigued during normal activity.	1 2 3 4
48.	I rely on over-the-counter pain relievers several times per week.	1 2 3 4
49.	My thinking is sometimes slow and fuzzy.	1 2 3 4
50.	I have difficulty concentrating.	1 2 3 4
51.	I'm nervous and anxious without knowing why.	1 2 3 4
52.	My mood swings from highs to lows.	1 2 3 4
53.	I often feel down or depressed.	1 2 3 4
54.	I'm fatigued or sleepy during the day.	1 2 3 4
55.	I'm often tired in the morning, even if I've slept well.	1 2 3 4

	QUESTION	ANSWER
56.	I suffer from apathy or lethargy.	1 2 3 4
57.	I get a cold or the flu multiple times per year.	1 2 3 4
58.	I experience frequent infections.	1 2 3 4
59.	My sensitivity to certain foods is getting worse.	1 2 3 4
60.	Being in a musty or moldy place makes me feel sick.	1 2 3 4
	Add up your scores to arrive at a rating for your level of Ama.	
	45 -55 Severe I 35-45 Moderate I 25-35 Mild I 11-25 Minimal	

HIGH AMA

If you scored between 45 and 55, your level of ama is high enough for you to notice symptoms daily. The toxic load in your body hasn't quite reached the crisis level, which is when you will start to experience disease, but you are edging closer to this point. Instead, it is creating a disruption in your ability to move, to think, to sleep, and to enjoy life's daily pleasures such as food. You may be more prone to seasonal illness and colds, and you are running down your immune system. This may have come from many years of eating a poor diet. Many people who need to lose 20 to 30 pounds are at this level of ama. And no matter what diet they try, nothing moves the number on the scale. You also have trouble with

For you, panchakarma will be the shock that your system needs to clear out the toxins and start fresh. Many patients at this level of ama report that they can't lose weight, don't feel strong enough to engage in a regular exercise routine, and are struggling with their emotions as well.

People at this level of ama are in a paradoxical situation. You absolutely need to detoxify your body, yet you can't just jump into a panchakarma treatment. First, you need to work to alleviate some of the strain on your body, to eat a modified diet and try on your own to remove some of the blockages in your system so that the treatments can be most beneficial. In the next chapter I'll discuss the pre-panchakarma regimen that you will need. Plan to begin this regimen at least a month before your scheduled treatment.

In addition, you should meet with your Ayurvedic practitioner a month before your treatment is set to begin in order to learn about any modifications for your diet and pre-treatment regimen. For example, those with a vata body type may need extra oils in their diet. They will also need to pay extra attention to meditative practices and sleep patterns before the treatment begins. Pitta and kapha types will need rigorous exercise and extra time sweating in a sauna to begin to move the excess toxins out of the body.

MODERATE AMA

If your score is between 35 and 45, you have a moderate level of ama. While your symptoms are nagging, they aren't actively interfering with your life every day. Perhaps you have occasional constipation or just one or two head colds per year. You are noticing a dip in your energy level in the mid afternoon on some days, while on other days you feel no appetite or a lack of energy. These fluctuations are what most people ignore before reoccurring symptoms manifest. The ama is building in your system, but this could be due to a temporary stressor in your life, or a bout of poor eating.

You are also a good candidate for panchakarma, even though you haven't reached the level of a health crisis. For you, the treatments will offer weight loss, rejuvenation, renewed energy, and better sleep. You will also become more resistant to stress and injury related to exercise.

For you, panchakarma still requires a preparation phase. Plan to meet with your practitioner at least two weeks ahead of your appointment to see if your body type requires alterations in the basic pre-treatment regimen. You should plan to be on the pre-treatment diet for two to three weeks before your first day of treatment. The pre-treatment diet will soften and remove some of your excess ama and get your body's tissues ready to dislodge the majority of excess ama in your system.

MILD AMA

If your score is between 25 and 35, you have a mild level of ama. This may be from ordinary toxins that can accumulate even if you have what's thought of as a healthy schedule and a healthy diet. There are still numerous ways in which toxins can sneak into your system, particularly if you eat at restaurants regularly. Even if you eat at healthy restaurants, you don't have complete control of your food chain. Your body is still functioning well, and you may be wondering if you are still a candidate for panchakarma.

For people with only a mild level of toxins, a panchakarma isn't necessary to prevent imminent disease. Yet it can still be beneficial to rejuvenate your body and make you feel your best. Many people who have worked to give themselves a healthy diet and those who have had panchakarma before, are probably in this category. In this case, your treatments may be more focused on rejuvenation and less on detoxifying your body.

Because you don't have a lot of toxins to remove, you may not need to modify your diet greatly in the weeks before your treatment begins. You will follow the prescribed diet, but may not feel that it is too taxing. You should be vigilant in your diet, avoid caffeine, alcohol and other indulgences while you wait for the panchakarma to begin. You will still need to do some of the preparations, including lubrication and internal cleansing to get the best result.

LOW AMA

If your score is between 11 and 25, Congratulations! You have a very low level of ama in your system. Many of my patients in this category have had panchakarma before, and stick to a rigorous Ayurvedic diet and schedule. They routinely work to make sure their doshas are balanced and that they get regular exercise which is appropriate for them. If you are in this category, you have few, if any, medical issues. You are probably already at or near a healthy weight and may already be in good shape.

People with low levels of ama will probably receive treatments that help rejuvenate the body rather than removing toxins.

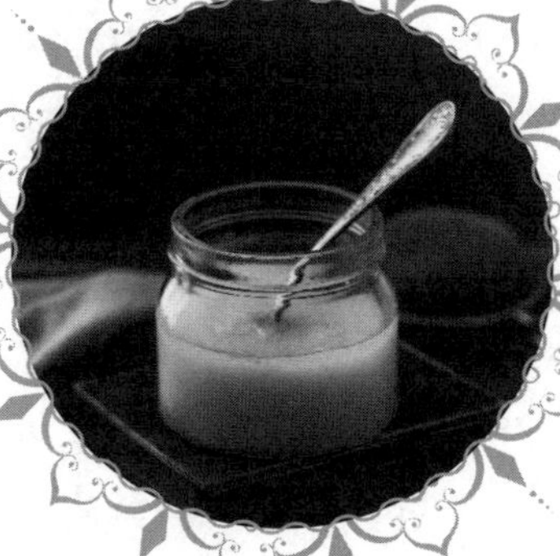

CHAPTER FOUR

PREPARATION FOR PANCHAKARMA

People sometimes believe that a panchakarma is a kind of spa treatment. They call us and try to book some dates. They want to know how much it costs and how many days they will need to stay near us. They think of this as a retreat.

In the Ayurvedic tradition, this is a medical treatment, not a vacation. That doesn't mean that the experience will be uncomfortable or painful. At many points it will feel nurturing and even spiritual. But you do have to take the preparation seriously. No one shows up for surgery with a full stomach. No one appears for a colonoscopy without having emptied their bowels. If you did this, the doctor would rightly send you home and re-schedule.

For Panchakarma, you have to prepare the body. This takes about a month. If you fail to take the preparations seriously, your practitioner might send you home to prepare properly. I've had people schedule the treatment with me and write down all of the instructions about how to adhere to a modified diet, how to do the two cleanses and how to start internal oleation. They are sincere in their promises to follow these directions. Then on the day of treatment, they come to the clinic and tell a story about having traveled during the month, having been distracted by work deadlines and so they didn't change their diet, didn't do any of the preparations or did them only sporadically. As a result, they have a body that is not ready for cleansing. In these cases, I absolutely tell people to reschedule.

If you show up to your treatment unprepared and your practitioner doesn't reschedule, you are likely to have a rough time with them. People come to my practice having had panchakarma somewhere else, where they didn't prepare, and they report serious headaches, or difficulty enduring the procedures. Some have an emotional crisis during the panchakarma itself and walk away from it feeling worse than before. The idea of the pre-treatment plan is to rid your body of some of the free flowing toxins in the digestive tract. When done correctly, this makes the actual panchakarma much more beneficial. You will sail through the procedures with a minimum of discomfort and walk away feeling better than you ever have.

The other benefit of these preparations is that you will feel wonderful, light, focused and energetic even before the treatments begin. Some patients call me about three weeks into their pre-panchakarma routine and say they don't need the treatments. That's how good they feel. We encourage our patients to go through with the treatments anyway because you are loosening a lot of ama in your tissues, and the treatments will clear this ama. We don't want it settling back into your cells and intestinal lining. We don't want it rushing back to your extremities. It's best to make a clean sweep of the body and start with newly cleansed organs and tissues.

The Preparatory Diet

The standard American diet leaves a lot of sludge in the digestive tract. If you look around you, you can probably see that most people consume coffee and a muffin or pastry for breakfast, followed by a deli sandwich and chips or soda for lunch, followed by a snack in the afternoon of crackers, candy or more coffee, followed by a late dinner of meat, starch and a cooked vegetable. This diet is rich in refined flours, sugar, and drinks that dry out the system, with hardly any fiber or nutrient-rich natural foods. Many of my new patients tell me that they eat nothing at all in the morning because they are still full from their late night meals. This is what happens when you consume a diet heavy in refined flours and overloaded with sugar and salt. The natural digestive fire gets snuffed out. Those who have switched to low carb or paleo or intermittent fasting diets can also succumb to eating lots of heavy meats and full fat dairy products. While it's great to be cautious of refined grains, baked goods and sugar, this diet isn't the answer for everyone. Some people can't safely consume large quantities of meats and heavy oils at every meal without slowing their digestion or feeling ill.

In addition, most people consume pre-packaged foods daily that are loaded with preservatives to give them a longer shelf life. The same chemicals that make these products shelf stable also make them harder to digest. This includes crackers, cookies, protein bars, breakfast cereals, and canned goods.

Most people don't eat enough fiber to cleanse their systems regularly. People also ingest pesticides and preservatives at an alarming rate. These, too, clog the system and get into your body, even at the cellular level. Plastics are everywhere, and these particles can enter your body and your blood stream in micro particles. Even if you eat cleanly, and rarely eat restaurant food and are very healthy, you'll want to eat foods that soothe and clear the digestive tract while you prepare for panchakarma. In addition, you want to build the micronutrients you need to feel healthy.

Here is the diet you should follow during the weeks before your treatment.	
Prioritize cooked vegetables	You can have steamed vegetables at every meal, including breakfast. You want to avoid salads and raw vegetables if possible, but you can have some greens in a morning smoothie if you like. People who love salads may balk at this, but raw vegetables take more energy to digest and we want to be letting your digestive tract working to rid itself of excess sludge. Think about stir frying vegetables or steaming them to get the bulk of your calories.
Eat a little less meat	You want to give up on the heaviest meats (such as beef, pork, and deli meats) during this phase. If you do eat meat, stick to fish and chicken, and only at the noon meal. Resist eating meat at the end of the day. You don't want to load up on meats at night when your digestion is weakening as it prepares for a natural overnight fast. My patients tell me that this one change has helped them sleep much better at night. They no longer suffer from indigestion or acid reflux.
Avoid dairy products	You don't need milk or cheese at this time. You can have a little bit of yogurt if you've made it yourself, but stay away from yogurt from the store as it contains lots of additives and sugars. You can turn to milks made from nuts such as coconut or almond if you feel you want to enjoy something creamy.
Eliminate wheat flour and most grains	Bread is the number one drug in the standard American diet. Many people eat bread or bread products at every meal. This is the time to shed all breads and all foods that contain wheat products that are difficult to digest and clog up the internal systems.

Here is the diet you should follow during the weeks before your treatment.	
Eliminate sugars, coffee, alcohol and other drugs	Yes, sugar is a drug and it produces a drag on your system. The same is true for coffee and alcohol. You want your body to be shrugging off dependence on these things while you prepare for treatment.
Enjoy nuts, nut butters and cold-pressed oils	Your body will need more healthy fats as you prepare to detox. This is the time to enjoy any of the nuts that you love and to dress your veggies with dressings made from fatty oils that will lubricate your system.
Use the spices recommended by your practitioner	Dress up your meals with spices that can help heat your system in winter or trigger mucus to be released from your system. For most people, spices help the body rid itself of ama. In some cases, depending on your body type, your practitioner may caution you against using excess spices.

When I outline this diet, some people rebel, asking how they can possibly adhere to this. If you rely heavily on fast food, restaurant food or frozen dinners for sustenance, this new diet will be a bit of a shock, but your body needs this change in order to reap the benefits of panchakarma.

People often argue that they eat the way they do because they are in a hurry. But it takes no more time to sauté a few greens in the morning (along with an egg or two) than it does to toast a bagel. The noon meal can be a hearty vegetable soup that also contains meat and rice. The evening meal is a stir fry or roasted vegetables with rice.

You may need to follow this diet for up to four weeks before your body is ready. But I have many patients who took a chance on this diet and never looked back. They lost weight almost immediately and felt such an increase of energy that they tell me they can't imagine eating any other way. Even if they returned to their regular diet for a few days, they noticed a decrease in energy levels, and more sluggish digestion. If you have a very low level of ama, you may notice that you are already eating fresh, healthy foods in abundance and might have the option of coming to treatment without altering your diet at all. Check with your practitioner.

MEAL TIMING

The Ayurvedic way of eating also notes that the timing of your meals is important. You want to be eating lightly in the morning. Consume your largest meal at noon and then eat lightly again at around 6:30. This will do wonders for your waistline, while improving the quality of your sleep. You need 10 to 12 hours of fasting time per day, which means that if you finish your evening meal at 7 or 7:30 at night and don't eat again until 6:30 the next morning, you are giving your digestive tract a well-earned break. This helps your body recover and get ready to take in nutrients. It will also help normalize fasting glucose levels, lipid profiles, and other metabolic measures.

HERBAL TEAS

Your practitioner may prescribe special teas for you to drink during the preparatory phase of treatment. At our clinic, we offer preparations that help with detoxification and weight loss. Other teas stimulate and clear the lymph system while reducing inflammation. Your practitioner will choose a tea for you based on your constitution. The tea given to you by your practitioner will contain important herbs such as coriander, fennel and cumin seeds, but it may also contain some mint, tulsi or other herbs that will gently pry loose the debris in your digestive tract. You will need to drink this tea each day for several weeks before treatment begins. Plan to make 2 quarts of this tea and keep it in a thermos or insulated water bottle near your desk. You can sip it slowly during the day and plan to finish by 4 p.m.

These teas also work to stimulate digestion, increase core body temperature, aid in weight loss, and the flavors help you to resist temptations to eat unhealthy foods. It curbs appetite naturally while also removing some toxins from the system.

SUPPLEMENTAL HERBS

Your practitioner may ask you to take special herbs depending upon your constitution, or your level of ama. The herbs you take will also depend on the season, your stress level, and your specific chronic health condition. These can be taken in pill form, powder, or even liquid. They usually include:

Triphala	This is known as the three fruits. It is made up of three different berries common in India and is one of the most popular Ayurvedic herbs. This has become so popular that you can find it in many drug stores and large chain supermarkets. It supports digestion and helps the bowels move more smoothly. It helps detoxify the body and supports the liver.

Trikatu	This contains three spices, including ginger, black pepper and long pepper. Together they stimulate the digestive system, the immune system and the respiratory tract. They support the circulatory system and warm the body.

EXERCISE

You will want to be generating a light sweat every day of this preparatory phase, and this means exercise. Sweat is the only eliminative function that gets rid of heavy metal toxicity. Most people will need to add daily exercise to their lives. Some of my clients already exercise and a few are very devoted to strenuous exercises, including weight lifting. I urge people not to lift weights as they prepare for panchakarma as it tends to sends toxins back into the deep tissues, while we want them coming to the surface in the form of sweat. You can walk every day or do some jogging. Yoga is an excellent form of exercise and if you can tolerate hot yoga, this is a great choice. Any form of exercise that brings you a light sweat will work as you prepare for treatment. If you have a body type that is somewhat sensitive to heat, your practitioner may recommend cooling activities, such as swimming. In other cases, you may need something more rigorous, such as hiking, biking, or traditional cardio exercises. All of these recommendations will be based on your level of ama and your body's natural constitution.

CASTOR OIL CLEANSE OR GH PILLS CLEANSE

Once or twice in the month before your treatment, you will want to empty your bowels completely. This will involve swallowing a tablespoon of castor oil in the morning instead of breakfast. You can mix it with some grapefruit juice if you don't like the taste. This is a laxative that will loosen your bowels. You'll need to pick a day in which you can stay near home and near the bathroom, because you will have to use the bathroom frequently.

After you take the castor oil, you may feel a little bit of cramping and some urgency to go to the bathroom. This should subside within four hours. Remember to eat only lightly for the rest of the day. You can have a little bone broth or clear soup at noon and a very light meal at dinner, maybe some steamed vegetables and herbal tea. You don't want to do any heavy exercise, but enjoy plenty of rest. You are taking care of your body by eliminating some of the ama that has been blocking your bowels from absorbing nutrients into your body. In the days after this cleanse you will feel lighter and more energetic.

Plan to do a castor oil cleanse twice before your treatment. Once about three weeks before, and another time about one week before. Don't try to do it more than twice. You don't want to deplete the body's nutrients or use laxatives to force weight loss. Instead, you are just giving your digestion a little boost to rid itself of some of the sludge that has accumulated.

While the goal of each castor oil cleanse is to promote four to five healthy bowel movements in a six hour window, it doesn't always work that way. I've had patients call me in a panic after taking the castor oil because nothing happened except for a little abdominal cramping. Or nothing happened for the first three to four hours and then they had a little bowel movement. They wonder if they should take it again, or double the dose. The answer is no. Your body is doing what it can.

Wait another 10 to 14 days and try for a castor oil cleanse for the second time. It usually works well the second time even if it doesn't work the first time.

In a few cases, people can't keep the castor oil down or it makes them nauseous. If this happens, contact your practitioner because there are herbs that work just as well but are easier for certain people to tolerate. We give these pills that contain castor oil plus some herbs.

INTERNAL LUBRICATION

In addition to your new diet and the castor oil cleanse, you'll want to increase the amount of oil in your diet. This means freely adding healthy oils to your diet in the form of nuts, and full fat salad dressings. You can use sesame oil, avocado oil or olive oil. You can add a little bit of coconut oil to your morning smoothie if you like.

We usually recommend that people eat ghee for about seven days before their treatment. Start with a single teaspoon of ghee. This is day one of internal oleation.

DAILY INTAKE OF GHEE							
DAY	1	2	3	4	5	6	7
GHEE	1 tsp	2 tsp	3 tps	4 tsp	5tsp	6 tsp	7 tsp

The next day, take two teaspoons of ghee. Don't worry about the fact that you are eating fats directly. This is the idea. Your body has stored toxins in the fats in your body, and you need to add fats to your digestive tract because they will help loosen the toxins lining your intestines and draw them out. Every day you increase your intake of oil by one tablespoon until the 7th day. On this day, you'll take in 7 teaspoons of ghee. It's important to take this oil on an empty stomach.

If you have a vata constitution, your body will love this part of the treatment. You may notice that your skin begins to glow. Your joints will creak less. Your muscles and tissues will drink in the oil and feel supple and healthy perhaps for the first time in a long time. People who need to lose weight or have a kapha constitution sometimes balk at taking in oils. All their lives they've been told to reduce their intake of fats and they fear that taking in several teaspoons of oil on an empty stomach will make them sick or cause them to gain lots of weight. My answer is that we need to lubricate the system before treatment. Any perception of weight gain will be reversed during treatment as the body gives up the toxins that are currently encased in body fat.

Not everyone lasts the full seven days. Some people begin to hate the dosage after three or four days. We sometimes get calls from patients saying that the oil makes them feel nauseous. One called to say that he couldn't take the final dose because the ghee began to repulse him. My advice in this case is to stop. Your body is giving you strong signals that it has enough oil and it is using that oil to capture toxins and repel them. Nausea is a strong sign that the toxins are beginning to flow and you don't need any more oil. People also notice that their skin is softer during this time. Your stools in the morning will contain some oil. You may have some gas. This is all fine. A few times, people have noted that when they get up in the morning, the normal discharge from their eyes is a little bit oily. None of this is harmful. The oils are seeping into your tissues and doing their work. Oil is a big part of panchakarma because it does such a good job of trapping and removing toxins. This internal oil cleanse is a big part of your preparation for the actual treatments to come.

EXTERNAL LUBRICATION (SELF MASSAGE)

You also want to apply oils to the skin. This will be most effective after you have been on your new diet for a week or so. By this time you will start to feel lighter, even if you haven't lost any weight. Don't worry about what the scale says. Once you feel lighter in your gut, your body is making important changes and your level of inflammation will decrease. This is the payoff for following this restrictive diet. Your body's natural level of inflammation will go down and your body will look and feel thinner. Now is the time to treat the body's largest organ—the skin—with lubricants to capture the toxins that your skin is shedding.

To do this, you can apply oils to your skin using self-massage. Then apply heat. In a way you are doing a panchakarma treatment for yourself. You can massage oils into your skin before you go on a morning walk and the natural sweat you exude during your walk will allow the oils to capture toxins coming out of the skin via exercise. You can also apply oils before going into a sauna and let the sweating in the sauna speed up your detox. Or, you can apply the oils all over your body before an evening shower or bath. My patients love this last option the best. It is such a relaxing way to end the day and they sleep like babies afterward. Even though it feels good, it's doing great work for your pre-detox plan.

The oils coat and soften the skin so that the heat in the water brings out the toxins more readily.

You don't have to do external oleation every day during your pre-treatment, but try to do it two or three times per week.

How You Will Feel

The patients I put on this protocol report that they feel better than they've ever felt before in their lives. Their new, clean diet makes their bowels happy. Their daily bout of light exercise fills them with energy. The internal and external oil treatments make their skin glow. They lose weight and gain focus in their daily lives. They sleep well at night and can bend and twist in new ways. This is what happens after three weeks with this new lifestyle.

That said, the first week can be a little rough, particularly if you have had an unhealthy diet for many years or if you have never exercised before. These are significant lifestyle changes. As your body begins to let go of some of the toxins in your digestive tract, you may feel a headache the first week or a little bit of fatigue or crankiness. You may find yourself feeling sad or dwelling on problems from the past. These are actually good signs that it's working. Your body is moving toxins out of the lining of the digestive system and out of the body. This is a process that involves the emotions as well as the body because the two are completely linked.

One of my patients really struggled with this new diet. She was used to eating lots of expensive cheeses at dinner and consuming an entire bottle of wine each day as well. She was heavily addicted to caffeine and routinely consumed three to four cups of coffee every day. All of these things were suddenly off the menu and her body rebelled. I think she called me every day of the first week, and wrote me daily emails about her headaches, her lethargy, her rashes and her anxiety. She had desperate food cravings. She had insomnia. I was able to reassure her that things would be okay if she stuck with it, which she did.

The only answer is to keep going, keep drinking the tea and exercising and it will all pass sometime in the first week. Most people experience these same sensations when they try to diet. I often feel that one of the big reasons people give up on dieting is because they feel the toxins release from the system and it's so unpleasant (if short lived) that they run back to old comforting habits. Also, many so-called diet foods don't contain enough fat or fiber to keep the bowels moving. What you should see after that first week is regular bowel movements. It might happen right away, but certainly in the first week you will be moving your bowels every day and that's the key to everything we are doing in this preparatory phase.

Your goal is to relieve your body of chronic indigestion. Any time you have trouble losing weight, it's because your body isn't digesting the food you take in. And so you are constantly hungry, constantly feeling empty. Good clean food, plenty of exercise and the right mixture of spices and oils will begin to reverse this. Once you have pushed through this first week, everything will get much better.

This is true even if you don't need to lose weight. I saw a man a few years ago who had no fat on his body. He had a very clean diet and exercised relentlessly, and as a result he looked emaciated. He surfed almost every day and swam in the ocean on the other days. He ran and biked almost every day. So, weight loss was not one of his problems. Instead, he'd been struggling with symptoms of adult-onset muscular dystrophy. He was having stiffness in his extremities and in his jaw. These things were interfering with his work because he would be seized with this stiffness and this muscle weakness during meetings at work to the extent that he sometimes struggled to talk. And he was having trouble exercising as well. He just couldn't move the way he wanted to, and was beginning to lose his balance at odd times of the day.

For the preparatory phase, we didn't have to change his diet at all, except to get him off the salads. Instead, he would be eating steamed vegetables. He had more of a vata-pitta constitution, so the daily swims in the cold water weren't helping him at all. I sent him to a yoga class instead where he could work on balance and stay warm while exercising. He needed a lot of internal oleation, so we saturated his diet with oils and had him massage even more oils into his skin. After the first two weeks, he called to say that he was finally sleeping well for the first time in his adult life. He felt less shaky and he had better control of his muscles.

When he came in for the panchakarma he had gained about 4 to 5 pounds, but he looked great. He had been so thin before but now his face was rounded and his skin glowed. He reported that he was able to balance on one leg again, which was quite a victory for him. He felt more in charge of his body and his movements. When we started the panchakarma, we knew he needed oil treatments more than anything. And we knew that when he went home, he needed those oils in his diet to keep his vata balanced. Now, he comes in once a year for treatment, and he calls it like taking his car in for and oil change. He has been symptom free for four years.

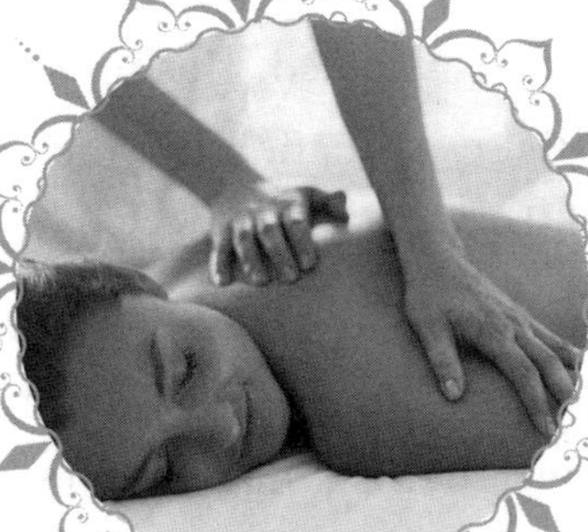

CHAPTER FIVE

WHAT IS POORVAKARMA?

Before we can eliminate toxins, we have to loosen them from the tissues in which they are embedded. This process must be tailored to you based on your initial examination by your practitioner. A skilled Ayurvedic clinician will examine you to determine the current state of your doshic imbalance by taking your pulse, looking at your tongue and asking you questions about your current state of health. Ideally, you have been following the diet and lifestyle prescribed to prepare your body for treatment. And now you are ready to begin the process of loosening the Ama in your body so that it can be eliminated through the digestive tract using the five Panchakarma treatments.

Amapachana

In the weeks before treatment begins, you should be given instructions on amapachana, which indicates the lifestyle changes that will begin to loosen ama in your body. These are detailed in an earlier chapter, but they should include removing heavy foods from your diet. Reduce the amount of meat you eat. Increase the fiber rich vegetables. Eliminate alcohol, nicotine and coffee. Eat your last meal earlier in the evening so that you have a longer period of fasting each night between dinner and breakfast. Your practitioner may prescribe specific herbs or herbal teas that will help your body remove the toxins in your digestive tract. This will make the panchakarma more effective. If you don't follow these instructions, there is a risk that the rest of the poorvakarma treatments will only increase the ama in your body. Your practitioner will give you instructions specific to your body type and to the calendar season. It's important to follow these instructions. Frequently people who make these lifestyle changes feel so good that their health symptoms abate before the treatment even begins. This is the important first phase of poorvakarma.

Snehana

The second phase of poorvakarma is snehana. This is a fancy term for saturating the body with herbal and medicated oils, both inside and out. Remember that oils are the primary means for loosening toxins and helping lift debris out of the tissues of the body, particularly the skin. I often use the analogy of the cooking pot. Suppose you oil a bowl thoroughly and then pour honey into it. The honey cannot stick to the bowl because the slippery quality of the oil does not allow it to. So the honey can be poured out of the bowl much more easily than if the bowl hadn't been oiled. Ama has the same sticky quality as honey, and so it moves easily after the body has been thoroughly oiled and relaxed with poorvakarma therapies.

Lipids form the membranes of every cell in your body. Introducing good, healthy oils to the body is itself cleansing and energizing. Because the skin is the body's largest organ, we can apply healing herbs directly to the skin and know that they will be absorbed into the body. The effect of this oil massage on the skin itself and on the psyche can be dramatic. People look and feel years younger, even after the first massage.

These medicated oils have been carefully prepared by your practitioner based on your body type and health concerns. We typically add 8 to 10 tablespoons of herbal powders to 4 cups of water and then boil the water down, strain it, and combine the resulting paste with one cup of oil. So, each cup of oil used in snehana can contain dozens of herbs in complex combinations. These activated herbs get massaged into your skin and so the body can absorb them without digesting or altering them. Through snehana, your body will absorb several tablespoons of healing herbs, and these will stay in your body for weeks after the Panchakarma has ended. This means that you will notice new healing results long after your treatment.

Some common herbs used in snehana include:	
ASHWAGANDHA	This herb relieves stress, improves energy levels, muscle tone and concentration. It can also help regulate blood sugar levels. It interacts powerfully with vata dosha, which means that it can help rebalance all three doshas.
BRAHMI	This herb boosts cognitive function while also reducing stress and bodily inflammation. It benefits a wide variety of bodily functions, including digestion, respiratory function and it improves skin tone. This herb also helps balance all three doshas.

Healing Massage

A big part of the snehana is the massage that comes with it, which is called abhyanga. The oils aren't merely spread over your skin, but massaged into the tissues using specific movements and hitting specific pressure points. These are known as marma points, and they often correspond roughly to those pressure points used in acupuncture in Traditional Chinese Medicine. There are 107 marma points on the body. But this type of massage is very different from the western style in which a single practitioner starts at the head and neck and works down toward the feet. In this traditional Ayurvedic massage, two practitioners will work together, one on either side of the body. They will be working to stroke the energy of the body in a particular direction and will be massaging these marma points in a specific order. This traditional massage isn't like anything you will have experienced before, and it's a crucial part of snehana.

In most cases, your practitioner will use sesame oil as the base for this massage. This oil works well with most body types. Those with a vata constitution or any vata disorders will find sesame oil to be tremendously soothing. In some cases, people suffer from traditional pitta disorders that cause excessive heat in the body. These may include certain skin conditions or hot flashes in menopause, or difficulty controlling anger. In this case, you may be treated with herbal coconut oil, which is much more cooling. Or your practitioner may choose to use cooling herbs to keep the body's equilibrium during the massage. For people with kapha disorders, your practitioner may choose mustard oil, which helps heat the body and improves metabolic functions. It also helps reduce inflammation and relieves joint pain.

Remember that snehana in Sanskrit can mean tenderness or love, and we often hold a client's hands before and after this treatment because it is both soothing and unsettling to be cared for in this way. The massage opens and releases the tensions at each of these marma points. Sometimes this also releases old memories and forgotten traumas. Some people experience a rush of love for someone they haven't thought of in years, and sometimes people experience complex and challenging emotions from the past. These marma points connect with the subtle body, which is a repository for memories and experiences. No matter what surfaces, this massage serves to clear and release old emotions and new insights.

In addition to this external oleation, you will be asked to take oil internally, usually ghee that has been infused with healing herbs. Ghee is essentially clarified butter. When butter has been cooked until the water evaporates, the resulting paste is edible and does not require refrigeration. On its own, ghee is an incredibly healthy substance and has been used as a staple of Ayurvedic healing for many centuries. Of all the saturated fats, this is the least saturated and it does not cause your blood cholesterol levels to rise. As a natural oil, it spreads easily through the tissues of the digestive tract and gets absorbed into the deeper tissues of the body. Ghee works on the body in a number of ways. It loosens and melts fat soluble toxins in the deeper tissues and in that sense, it works like soap and water to cleanse the body. At the same time, it helps lubricate all of the internal tissues. Many modern substances and lifestyle choices have a drying effect on the body, and this oleation helps to restore natural suppleness to the internal tissues and organs.

While it's traditional to use ghee for internal oleation, your practitioner may choose sesame oil, which also works well for certain body types.

Swedana

After your massage, you will go directly to the final phase of poorvakarma, which is heat therapy. Swedana literally means "sweat" and that's pretty much the goal of this treatment. During massage, your body is beginning to absorb the oils and herbs. By adding heat, we open the pores and channels of the body to allow the oils to spread even deeper into your tissues.

Some people are resistant to the idea of heat at first. I have patients who tell me that they can't tolerate hot yoga or hot weather and they don't want to do the steam treatment. I have to explain that the oil they've swallowed will help them to tolerate the heat. In fact, you should probably take a little bit of ghee before you go to a hot yoga class, because that will increase the cleansing action of the yoga poses. It will also help you to tolerate the heat a little bit better. Also, a yoga class can last 90 minutes, while this steam treatment will probably last no longer than 20 minutes. Your practitioner will do several things to improve your comfort. Because the head and neck must be kept cool, you will probably have cool cloths placed on your head or face. While the body will be sweating, your head will remain cool, and this helps people to tolerate the treatment better. Of course, my patients with a vata constitution love the steam heat and heat of any kind. It can actually take them longer to work up a sweat in any situation because their bodies absorb so much heat.

There are several ways to apply steam heat to the body. The most common is called bashpa swedana. This applies steam heat evenly to the whole body (except the head and neck). You will sit inside a sweatbox or steam chamber with only your head exposed. Your practitioner will keep your head cool with cold compresses. You will spend maybe 15 to 30 minutes just sitting quietly and sweating. In some cases, you might be wrapped in a cotton sheet that can help absorb the sweat and oils.

Afterward, you will be able to wipe yourself down with a towel. Your practitioner may apply therapeutic poultices or pastes to select areas to further detox specific body parts. In many cases, you will be advised to take a bath in lukewarm water. If the heat becomes a little bit taxing, your practitioner may use cooling or astringent substances on the skin to quickly cool you down. Cool drinks will also help reduce the body's temperature if needed.

A second type of treatment is called nadi swedana, which means applying steam heat to a specific part of the body. Nadi means "channel" or a tube. In this case it pumps steam so that it can be applied locally. This wet heat penetrates more deeply in areas such as the lower back or certain joints that may be stiff or sore. These localized treatments last between five and seven minutes. Sometimes your practitioner may want to apply steam heat to your face as part of a treatment.

There are many types of swedana therapy that might be used during your panchakarma treatments. Your practitioner may encourage you to exercise to the point of sweating. You might be asked to wear heavy jackets or cover yourself with warm blankets. You might be given spicy foods to eat that will provoke a little bit of flushing or sweating. You will probably receive many types of thermal treatments because heat is often very healing. You might be asked to take a hot bath and put some herbs in the water, or you might use a heating pad to target a specific area. Rest assured these treatments have been tailored to you and your body's needs.

Shirodhara

There is an additional poorvakarma treatment that is sometimes done before the main therapies. It offers an emotional cleanse through deep relaxation. Shirodhara is a subtle and profound treatment of pouring warm oil in a slow, steady stream on the forehead. It calms and nourishes the central nervous system and promotes tranquility. The idea is that only through deep relaxation can we overcome deeply rooted imbalances. Many patients have reported that they experience altered states of consciousness during this treatment. Some people recall highly specific memories that were once lost to them. Others say that they are filled with gratitude and love.

This is one Ayurvedic treatment that has captured the attention of several researchers in Japan who asked healthy female volunteers to undergo a Shirodhara treatment outside of panchakarma. They wanted to measure the effects of this treatment and they didn't even want an attendant present to control the flow of oil in case the presence of another person might be influencing the experiences of participants. So they designed a robot that would control the flow of oil on their volunteers. The control group was asked to lie down on a massage table and relax for 30 minutes while the study group did the same but enjoyed the oil treatment. The study reported that the subjects who underwent this modified Shirodhara experienced significant reduction in anxiety and an increase in altered states of consciousness according to physiological and biochemical markers measured during the study.[1]

I can attest that many people slip into altered states during this procedure. For most of them, these states provide new insights as well as a sense of wellbeing. Only once did a patient experience something he felt was upsetting. This man was going through the first day of his first panchakarma. During the Shirodhara, he jumped up alarmed and tried to rush out of the clinic. I caught up to him and persuaded him to return, but he was quite agitated. When we were able to talk more he said that he had a vision of his father, who had died years before. This man had had no relationship with his father as an adult because the father had been so abusive to him. At one point, the father had even taken out a gun and threatened his life. Although this was extremely traumatic at the time, the patient cut his father out of his life, and then forgot about it for the most part and moved on as best he could. During the Shirodhara, the warm oil relaxed his senses and opened his consciousness enough that he had the sense of his father standing next to him. In fact, he had the feeling that his father's hand was stroking his head in that loving way that a parent would for a resting child. He found this idea of a loving, nurturing father so jarring that he didn't want to continue with treatment. I talked to him about how this could be a healing experience for him, a way toward a new level of self-actualization. But he kept saying, "I felt him there. I know he was there." Eventually, he did return to finish his Shirodhara and the rest of his panchakarma treatment. The image of his father never returned, but at the end of the week, this patient agreed that he'd reached a level

1. Uebaba et. al. Psychoneuroimmunologic effects of Ayurvedic oil-dripping treatment. J Altern Compliment Med, 2008, Dec. 14(10):1189-98.

of calm self-assurance that he'd never had before.

These three procedures together work to pull the physical and emotional toxins out of the deep tissues of the body and deposit them into the gastrointestinal tract. Then you are ready to undergo the main procedures of panchakarma, which are designed to eliminate them from the body entirely. These three poorvakarma procedures will likely be repeated every day of your treatment regimen. Each day that you go through them will be slightly different and your experience with them will likely deepen as you go. Each day, your practitioner will re-evaluate your health and may make modifications to these for maximum benefit.

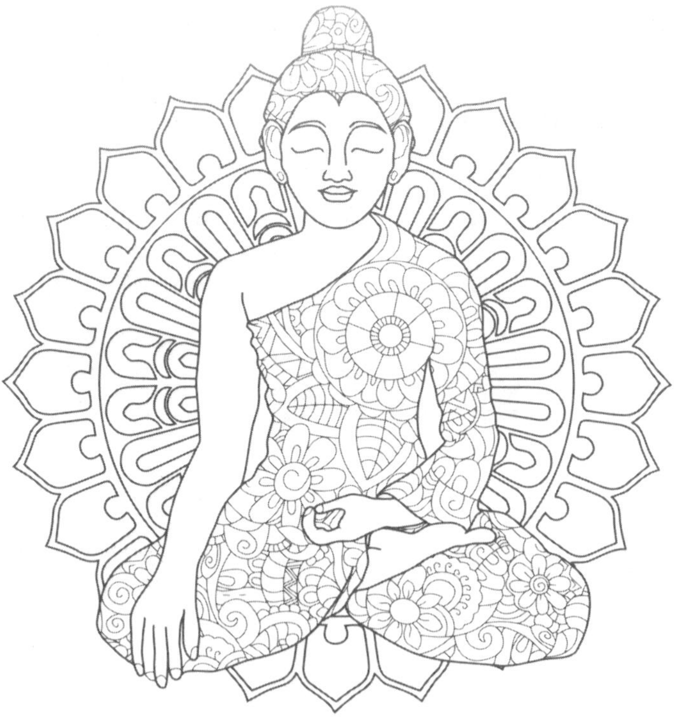

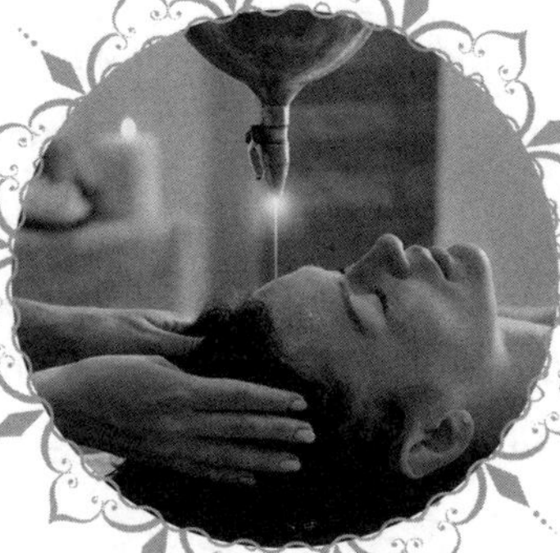

CHAPTER SIX

WHAT IS PRADHANKARMA?

At last you are ready for the main treatments of panchakarma. For these, you will come to the clinic every day for several days in a row to receive the treatments designed for you. Every patient will have a regimen designed for them based on the person's constitution, age, physical strength and the specific doshic imbalances to be addressed. These treatments are also tailored to the season in which the treatment is taking place because your body has different needs and different challenges throughout the year.

This treatment plan includes the number and type of treatments to receive each day as well as their exact sequence and duration. It's a little bit different for everyone, but rest assured that the doctor will be meeting with you daily to take your pulse, discuss your progress, answer your questions and adjust the treatment regimen as needed. Most people will receive some kind of enema (basti) every day, some type of massage (snehana) with oils or milk or buttermilk, or perhaps a scrub, and some type of warming treatment (swedana).

Your doctor will also prescribe a specific daily routine for you. I've included an example schedule below. Note that the schedule has set times for meals, for gentle exercise, for meditation and for rest and reflection. We discourage people from vigorous exercise during the treatment regimen, and we ask patients to put away all electronic devices. This is no time to be mindlessly pounding away on a treadmill or zoning out in front of a television or iPad. You need all of your senses focused on the body and the transformation that is happening in your body and in your mindset.

A Typical Day in Panchakarma

TIME	ACTIVITY
7 to 8 a.m.	Yoga, exercise or morning walk
8 a.m.	Breakfast
9 a.m. to noon	Treatments
Noon	Lunch with herbal tea
1 to 2 p.m.	Consult with the doctor
2 to 4 p.m.	Beach walk, writing, reading
4 to 6 p.m.	Meditation, yoga or beach walk
6 to 7 p.m.	Light dinner
7 to 9 p.m.	Reading, drawing or light activity
9 to 10 p.m.	Bedtime

Classical Panchakarma vs Kerala Style

In a classical panchakarma,
patients receive five main treatments, including:

VAMANA (vomiting)	**VIRECHANA** (purging)	**BASTI** (oil enema)
NASYA (nasal irrigation)	**RAKTAMOKSHANA** (bloodletting)	

These treatments will be described in detail in the following chapters. It's important to know that these classical treatments are based upon Vedic writings and are the most intense and transformative treatments. However, because of US laws, practitioners have some limitations on these treatments. Specifically, we cannot induce vomiting or draw blood from patients in an Ayurvedic clinic. These procedures are reserved for medical professionals.

This doesn't mean that you will be receiving a watered down version of Ayurvedic treatments. What it means is that your practitioner will rely on supplemental treatments from the Kerala style of panchakarma. Kerala is a state on the southwestern coast of India, and it is known as a vibrant center for Ayurvedic clinics. It has a mild climate and an abundance of the medicinal herbs used in Ayurveda. The Kerala style of Ayurveda considers the skin to be the primary organ of the body. Practitioners in Kerala have developed a number of supplemental treatments to introduce healing herbs into the body through the skin. That's why a US-based clinic may rely more on massages, scrubs, heat and drops for the nose, eyes and ears as part of your daily treatment. These treatments are very powerful on their own, and long tradition has shown that these skin-based techniques are effective in detoxing the system and reversing disease. Your practitioner will explain the prescribed supplemental treatments and how they will work for you.

Common Supplemental Treatments

PINDA SWEDA (RICE BOLUSES)

This is an effective rejuvenation therapy that nourishes and stimulates the skin. A special type of rice is cooked with medicinal herbs. The infused rice is tied up into a bolus (pottali), then dipped in an herbal decoction mixed with warm milk. This is what the practitioners will use to vigorously massage your body. This procedure drains toxins from the skin while nourishing the tissues. This improves blood circulation, skin tone and muscle tone. It also relieves joint pain and calms the nervous system.

VALUKA POTTALI (SAND BAG)

The word Valuka means sand in Sanskrit. In this treatment, cheese cloths are filled with medicated sand and then tied into boluses. Once heated, these boluses are used to all over body for massage.

This treatment helps for joint pains and stiffness. This treatment is done usually followed by an oil massage.

TAKRA DHARA (HERBAL BUTTERMILK)

This treatment is just like Shirodhara except it uses buttermilk instead of oil. This treatment involves using medicated warm buttermilk that is poured over the forehead in a slow continuous stream. Buttermilk is cooling and cleansing. It cools the body, which is good for pitta. Takes out heat, anger from head, relaxes the mind and balances the nervous system.

KSHEER DHARA (HERBAL MILK)

This treatment involves pouring medicated milk that has been warmed slightly over the body temperature. It can be poured over the forehead, just as with Shirodhara, this treatment is both cooling and nourishing, making it great for pitta and vata imbalances.

KASHAYA DHARA (HERBAL DECOCTION)

Herbal concoction can also be used for Shirodhara. it is indicated for people with any skin, hair or scalp condition. It's also good to relieve headaches, and pitta imbalances in general.

UDVARTANA (EXFOLIATING SCRUB)

This powerful detoxifying treatment made from herbs that have been slightly moistened by sesame oil. The herbal paste is scrubbed over the entire body. This scrubbing action invigorates the skin and muscles while helping to cleanse the lymphatic system. It also improves circulation. This treatment is often followed by an herbalized steam bath (Swedana) on a tented massage table. This heat treatment further allows the skin to shed toxins while also allowing you to sink into deep relaxation.

MARMA MASSAGE

This Ayurvedic massage is often part of the panchakarma treatment, but sometimes patients request this type of massage on its own because it is both calming and stimulating. This involves a coordinated massage from two practitioners working in tandem on each of the body's 108 marma points, which are junctions of the mind, body and spirit. The combination of oil, heat and pressure regulates the flow of prana through the energetic pathways in the body. It also clears emotional toxicity and improves emotional wellbeing.

NETRA BASTI (EYE BATH)

Netra basti is a restorative and preventative Ayurvedic treatment for the eyes. Your practitioner will fashion a dough from flour and spices and build a dam around your eyes. This dam will be filled with herbal ghee. You will be directed to do eye exercises while immersed in the ghee. This helps to improve eyesight and reduces dryness and itching in the eyes. This treatment is often given along with marma points massage and a foot massage with a kanse bowl, which is rounded at the end and made from special healing metals. The foot massage stimulates certain points in the foot that correspond to the eyes and further enhance the rejuvenating qualities of the basti.

Possible Complications

Many of the treatments in panchakarma may sound a bit like spa treatments, but it's important not to underestimate the effect that they will have on the body and mind. That's why you should always undergo panchakarma treatments under the supervision of an Ayurvedic physician. Think of this as a medical treatment, one that is every bit as serious as a surgery.

Patients are taking real risks if they fail to prepare their bodies for treatment in the way the doctor has prescribed or if they break with the daily routine and diet prescribed for them during treatment. You don't want to bring your body to these main treatments if you haven't prepared adequately. If the treatments commence on someone who is not prepared, the patient can experience headaches, lethargy, and emotional turmoil that is difficult to reverse. Likewise, if you ingest a toxic diet during the main treatments, you are risking real complications. These include fever, insomnia, headaches, confusion and anxiety, and sometimes delusional thinking. It's important to follow your doctor's advice before, during and after treatment so that you can experience the maximum benefits and avoid any complications. If you do experience any negative side effects from a treatment, be sure to speak to your physician so that the remaining treatments can be altered accordingly.

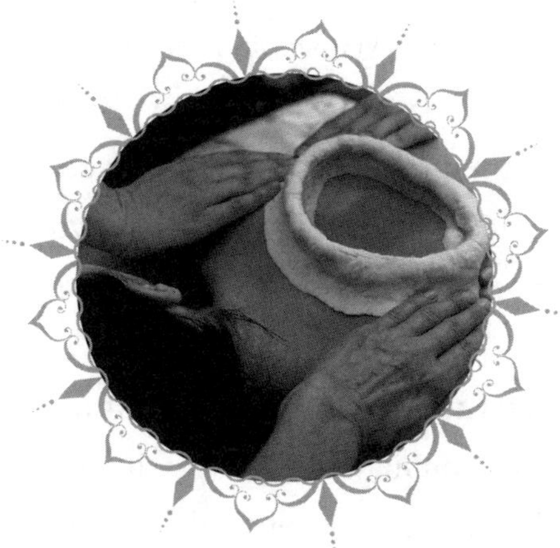

CHAPTER SEVEN

BASTI

The basti is an ancient Ayurvedic treatment that can be used for many things. The word "basti" means urinary bladder. In the old days, a doctor would use the preserved bladder of a cow or sheep as a sort of bag to hold medicated oils or water. They would then connect a wooden or metal nozzle to it and use this to push the medicines and fluid into the colon.

People often refer to this as an enema, but it's very different from the traditional enemas you may be familiar with. In a traditional enema, the goal is to flush the colon or part of the colon to clear out feces. And this is considered a type of cleansing. But most of the time, the enema floods the colon with fluids, which causes immediate cramping and an urgent, uncomfortable rush to the bathroom. You won't have any of these uncomfortable feelings during a basti treatment. While an enema is useful for the simple cure of constipation, it doesn't provide secondary medical benefits. In fact, repeated enemas with water can dry the membranes of the colon and can actually damage them.

Basti, by contrast, uses far less fluid. Instead, it introduces healing herbs and oils into the colon, so that they can be absorbed into the body's other tissues. When you receive a basti, you will not feel an immediate or distressing urge to produce stool. Instead, you will be allowed to relax as the fluids and herbs are slowly introduced to the colon and you will keep the medicine inside for a time to let them work.

This is such a powerful treatment that it can even work wonders on someone who is not getting a full panchakarma treatment. I had one patient came to me after he had suffered a terrible skateboarding accident. He had back injuries and chronic pain for which he took opioid medications. He had been on these medications for several weeks and although he was able to reduce the dosages, he had terrible constipation and pain in his bowels. Many pharmaceuticals have the side effect of drying out the body's tissues and opioid medication is well known to cause constipation because it tends to halt the body's digestive movement. The nerves that signal the contraction of digestive muscles seize up, and this can cause both nausea and constipation. These side effects can last for weeks after you stop taking these drugs. The patient came to me because of this severe constipation and asked for herbal laxatives because the over-the-counter laxatives he had tried didn't work. I told him that we had to go after the root problem more directly.

With some reluctance, he agreed to weekly basti treatments until we could resolve the problem. He was also ready to give up the opioid entirely. I gave him oil herbal basti with a little bit of salt to help the body absorb the oils. The first two times we gave him oil, he had good pain relief, but no bowel movements at all. Not a single drop of oil came out. The third time, his body was back to normal. We gave him some exercises to do in water to strengthen his back muscles, some specific stretches and some healing herbs. And he was able to give up all of his pain medications and felt great. A couple of months later he came back for a full panchakarma.

Who Benefits from Basti

Anyone who suffers from any kind of pain can benefit from lubricating the colon. It's good for any vata disorders, because these tend to create or mimic pain in the body.

Many times, patients come for a panchakarma because they have migraines, neck pain, joint pain or tendonitis, difficulties with concentration or anxiety. They sometimes ask directly, "Why are you giving me an enema? My health concerns have nothing to do with my colon." But everything in your body has to do with the colon and how it is functioning. In Ayurveda, we know that digestion is the foundation of good health. A primary means of assessing good health is looking at what the colon is producing each day. In addition, the colon doesn't merely store and move waste products, it also absorbs nutrients into the body. When we flush the colon with a mixture of water and medicated oils, we are allowing those medicines and healing oils to move directly into the other tissues in the body.

Any vata imbalance has to be dealt with through the colon, which is the primary organ that affects the vata dosha. Because vata energy is the energy of movement, any disorder that has to do with physiology, the nervous system or the joints is probably due to a vata imbalance. So is insomnia, and people often report that the basti treatment allows them to get to sleep easily at night. It allows them to relax, rids them of scattered thinking. And it really does improve cognitive functioning. It literally grounds you.

According to the traditional texts, there is also a strong connection between the lining of the colon and the health of the bones in someone's body. And it's true that many people who suffer from irritable bowel syndrome are at a higher risk for developing osteoporosis or joint pain. It's thought that disorders such as IBS, Crohn's and even celiac disease interfere with the body's ability to absorb the nutrients to feed the bones properly. By nourishing, softening and opening the lining of the colon with oil, you are protecting your entire skeletal system.

Anyone who can't use Vamana or Virechana because they are too weak can still benefit from the cleansing action of basti. A combination of bastis can be used instead.

Basti should be avoided for those who have diarrhea, rectal bleeding, ulcerative colitis, diverticulitis, colon cancer, external hemorrhoids or polyps.

Types of Basti

There are many different types of basti. Some are primarily water based, others use oil. In rare cases, practitioners may use other substances, including beet juice. This is called a bruhana basti. In cases where the digestive fire is very weak, a practitioner may use pureed vegetables that have been well cooked and cooled as the medium for a basti. These allow nutrients to enter the colon directly.

Most panchakarma treatments use either medicated oils or medicated water with a little bit of oil as the method for cleansing and nourishing the colon and balancing the vata dosha.

NIRUHA BASTI

This is a more cleansing basti, in that it helps flush toxins directly from the colon. Most of the liquid is water, but some oil can be added to this in addition to the medicines. The treatment uses less than 2 cups of liquid. The liquid is administered slowly, so as not to provoke the colon to expel the fluids. You won't need to void the colon immediately after the basti is administered. Instead, you will be encouraged to hold the liquid in for a little less than an hour before letting it go. This won't be uncomfortable at all. Instead, you will be able to feel the relaxing effects of the treatment. You may receive one of these for several days in a row, and this allows for deeper cleansing of the tissues.

In some rare cases, people with extremely dry tissues in the colon can't produce stool after the basti treatment. This is because the dry colon absorbs so much of the liquid that the practitioner has to administer a second basti, mostly made up of oils, to get the colon moving again.

ANUVASAN BASTI

This is much more of a nourishing treatment. Most of the liquid used is medicated oils that seep into the colon and surrounding tissues in order to heal and strengthen them. These are usually given after a course of cleansing bastis. And these require less liquid and are meant to be retained in the body for a longer period of time, even overnight. This type of basti is administered slowly in order to allow the oils to work gently on the colon.

Some Ayurvedic hospitals administer a very slow version of this technique using an IV drip. This allows the oils to seep into the colon a few drops at a time. Most clinics that offer panchakarma don't do this because it can take an hour or longer to administer the oils.

Different types of oils can be used in an internal basti, but the most common is sesame oil. The oil is very carefully infused with specific herbs. While there can be hundreds of different herbal combinations, the most common are Triphala, which contains three different kinds of dried fruits. When used in combination, these berries have a very healing effect on the lining of the colon. Many people take Triphala orally to improve digestion and intestinal functioning. Ashwagandha is another herb that heals the colon and can also be taken orally to calm the nervous system and strengthen energy levels. When used in a basti, it has much more powerful and immediate effects. Shatavari can help women with many conditions, including balancing the hormones and regulating menstruation. Sometimes basti oils will contain dozens of different combinations of herbs.

The process of introducing an herb to oil takes tremendous time and patience. The herbs are boiled in water to reduce them to concentrate, then added to the oil and boiled further to reduce the remaining water. This process is repeated for each additional herb in a process that can take months. The final preparation contains high potency herbs in great concentration. This process is called curation.

How Basti is Administered

Basti is administered after several days of poorvakarma treatments. It is the payoff for all of this preparation. The internal and external oleation combined with massage loosens the ama in the tissues and delivers it into the digestive tract. The steam treatments further facilitate the release of ama all over the body. Some of this ama is excreted via sweat glands through the skin. The rest goes into the digestive tract. A practitioner will use an enema bag or a bulb with warmed oil that has been infused with herbs to gently introduce the medicated oils or water into your colon. It's usually painless and often relaxing. As the medicines begin to work, you may feel a sense of wellbeing come over you and may drop into a meditative state. Your practitioner may give you a hot water bottle to put on your abdomen. The warmth will help your body to absorb the oils and medicine and it will improve circulation in that area as well. You may be given a liner for your underwear before you get up from the table. This will absorb any little bit of oil that may escape as you go about your day.

Occasionally, people will experience a little bit of cramping. This usually indicates that there is some dried waste in the colon. The cramping will pass as the colon absorbs the oils and the toxins begin to loosen. It's far more common for people to feel relaxed as though they've just meditated. The oils inside the colon have an immediate effect on the vata dosha and the entire nervous system and this effect lasts for hours and days afterward.

After these basti treatments, you will be encouraged to keep track of your bowel movements as you may have more than one after treatment. These bowel movements may be oily and soft or be made up mostly of oil at first. Occasionally people have no bowel movements or urge to use the bathroom after a first basti. If this happens, it may be that your colon tissues were so dry that they absorbed all of the oils like blotting paper. That generally indicates that your body really needed this treatment. A subsequent treatment will likely produce a bowel movement.

Your practitioner may alternate between these cleansing and nourishing treatments. And he or she will talk to you and observe how you are responding to these treatments in order to adjust the ingredients in the herbal preparations. Each one of these treatments is loosening the toxins that have settled into your colon during the poorvakarma. While you may feel relaxed, your body is doing a lot of work to remove its toxic load. You may feel tired after a basti and even more so during a series of basti treatments, so make sure to get plenty of rest. Your energy level will rebound after the panchakarma treatment ends.

Topical Basti

Basti can also refer to the application of a pool of oil to a specific body part to encourage healing and detoxification in that area. For this, the practitioner will make a paste or dough out of black gram flour. And build a dam around a part of the body that will hold a pool of oil. While you rest, the medicated oils will seep directly into the skin and tissues of that body part. So, if you are struggling with sore knees, you might have an external basti on each knee. Some people benefit from a lower back basti (although an internal basti will also help alleviate back pain and spasms). This type of treatment can even help with emotional issues. I've used an external basti over the heart. This is not really to treat heart disease. Rather, it focuses medicine and lubrication over the heart marma point, which is also the heart chakra. Those who have energy trapped at this point, and for those who are stuck in grief. A practitioner can even create such a dam over the top of your head, which will help clear the senses and improves your general energy level.

We even do this type of basti to help improve eyesight. We call this a netra basti. I had a 75-year-old patient who had experienced blurriness in her vision lately. She had some digestive and metabolic issues as well, which is common among people her age. However, her real concern was her blurry vision. She had been scheduled to go renew her driver's license and feared that she wouldn't be able to pass the eye test and retain her license. She came in for a netra basti each week for four weeks. We built a dough dam around her eyes and poured in the medicated ghee. She would rest like that for up to 20 minutes and then we remove the dam, wipe away the oil and stimulate certain marma points on the face. The oil provides soothing and lubrication for the eye and the muscles and tissues around the eye, and these are most responsible for helping you to focus. We supplemented this with a few drops of oil in the nose, because you want all of these sensory tissues to stay lubricated as you age. After four weeks, she noticed how much her eyesight improved and later told me that she sailed through her eye test with flying colors.

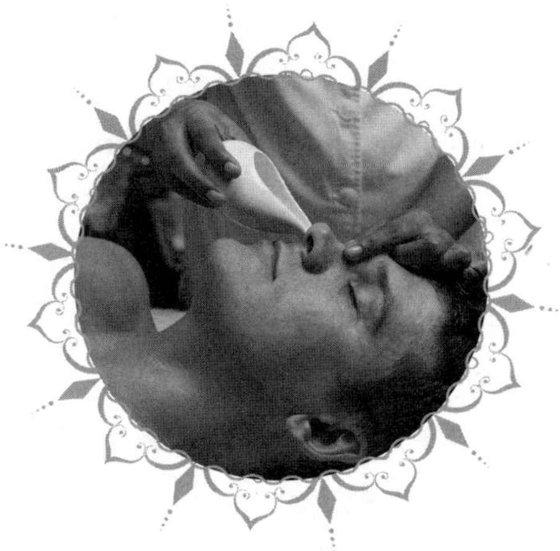

CHAPTER EIGHT

NASYA

The nose is the doorway to your brain and nervous system. Whatever you inhale, you take directly into your brain. This is the portal through which pollutants, viruses and other impurities can enter your body. Remember that all of your senses are centered on or around your face and they are all connected. A spring cold won't just clog your nose, but will also block the ears, block the taste buds, create discharge in the eyes and create fogginess in your mind. By contrast, anything you do to strengthen and protect your nasal passages will help your hearing, taste, sight and mental clarity.

In classical Ayurvedic texts, the nose is not just the doorway to the brain, but it also conducts the prana vata, the seat of knowledge, perception and spiritual awareness. Nasya won't merely cleanse these tissues. It also has the power to awaken a higher consciousness. All of your negative sensations come with emotional toxins as well. These remain and reside in the head and neck. Nasya is the way to remove them all.

At the same time, the tissues inside the nostrils and sinuses are delicate and must be treated carefully. You'll find this treatment to be soothing, relaxing and gentle. In fact, it's one of the only panchakarma treatments that many patients can do at home. In fact, you can do it on a daily basis. During the spring season, many people experience allergies and congestion. They've just experienced the dry winter season that puts stress on the nasal passages. Then the spring moisture arrives and they find themselves susceptible to colds. When the pollen season begins, these tissues become even more inflamed. An easy preventative measure is to warm a little bit of sesame oil and massage the oil inside your nose. Tilt your head back and inhale the oil so that it spreads throughout the nasal cavity. Do this a couple of times a day during the dry season. You should do it before you go out on a very cold, dry day. This will help protect your sinuses from bacteria and pollution. You can even put a couple of drops of oil directly into your nose before you go to sleep. Many times, my patients have been cured of snoring from this simple daily habit. They keep the oil next to their beds. As an alternative, you can apply a little bit of ghee to your nostrils. It helps sharpen the senses. The nostrils and the back of the throat serves as the nexus of all the senses.

When the treatment is used as part of panchakarma, it is much more involved, and therefore more beneficial.

Who Benefits from Nasya

This treatment benefits anyone with problems relating to the head, the senses or the nervous system. It relieves migraines and headaches, jaw pain, toothaches, sinusitis, or stiffness in the neck and shoulders. Cleansing and nourishing the nasal passages will also lift the mood and settle the nervous system. This benefits anyone suffering from depression, anxiety and many other mental health issues. Those with a longstanding kapha disorder who routinely suffer from congestion, excess mucus, allergies or lethargy will find relief with this treatment. Others have chronically dry sinuses and eyes. This will help relieve those symptoms as well. A lot of people suffer from sleep apnea, and we've had patients give up their C-PAP machines after experiencing a Nasya treatment if they continue to use oil drops at home. Some patients have told us that they noticed an improvement in their eyesight because of Nasya.

I had a patient who had persistent congestion in his nose and sinuses. He snored at night and had trouble sleeping because his congestion got so much worse at night. Things became so frustrating for him that he went to a specialist who told the patient that he had nasal polyps and the only cure was surgery. He came to me because he was hoping to put off surgery for as long as possible. I wasn't so sure that the diagnosis was correct, but I had no way to know until we calmed down his nasal passages. Sometimes swelling and inflammation from toxicity can look worse than it is. I put him on a clean diet with lots of fruits and vegetables and very little dairy. And told him to eat less at dinner and to eat earlier in the evening. I gave him nose drops to use each night, then brought him in to the clinic for a Nasya treatment. He received a massage with herbal oils over the head, face and neck, then he inhaled herbal steam. Then he went home but continued to eat well and use the nose drops each night. Within two weeks, he had stopped snoring entirely and his nasal passages were clearer than they had been in a long time. Not only that, he'd lost a little weight and felt that his energy was soaring. After a month, he felt totally normal, but he still feared that he needed surgery. He was afraid to go against his doctor's diagnosis. I told him to stick with it for another month and then go back to the doctor for a second evaluation. That following evaluation showed no evidence of polyps and the surgeon changed his diagnosis. It's possible that this man never had polyps at all. Instead, the swelling inside his nose was so severe, it looked like polyps.

Putting drops in the nose is an amazing form of Nasya that you can do at home. One of my patients is a professional singer who had trouble with a dry, scratchy throat. She came in for a single Nasya treatment and felt amazing afterward. Now she gives herself nose drops at home every night along with gargling with warm water with a little honey, turmeric and salt. She says that without these daily habits she wouldn't be able to sing. She sleeps better at night and wakes up energized every day.

Having said that, there are some conditions in which you should not do this on your own at home. It's not a good idea to use nasal oil drops while you are pregnant or menstruating. If you are experiencing shortness of breath or exhaustion from exercise, you don't want to clog the nose for any reason. For the same reason it's also not good for the elderly or very small children. You also shouldn't do this immediately following a meal, a bath, exercise, sex, or after drinking alcohol. Give the body a chance to recover from exertion before trying Nasya at home. You should be relaxed and calm.

Types of Nasya

Because the nasal passages are delicate and because they link all of the senses, there are various ways to treat them using Nasya. In some cases, patients may need to have a treatment that can extract the accumulated toxins that have been causing chronic congestion. In other cases, we need to nourish and rejuvenate tissues that have become dry and irritated. Finally, some patients respond to the many palliative effects of Nasya, even though they don't have congestion. This form of treatment has a calming effect on the nervous system as a whole.

SHODHANA NASYA (CLEANSING)

This is an oil-based treatment. Oils infused with herbs are dripped into the nasal cavity where the tissues can absorb both the oil and the medicine. This helps cleanse the tissues and clears the senses. The herbs used in this treatment increase secretions in the nasal passages to help remove toxins. This has the effect of relieving chronic headaches, sinus congestion or a feeling of overall heaviness in the senses. This is usually administered with strong, pungent herbs. Many practitioners use Gotu Kola, which is known for its calming influence on the nervous system. Others use Eucalyptus. Sometimes they may even use the common black pepper, which can clear out excess mucus in the sinuses.

BRUHANA NASYA (REJUVENATING)

This is also oil based, usually ghee infused with healing herbs. And this treatment is more nourishing in nature. It will not remove blockages and heaviness, but instead soothes the sinuses and calms the nervous system, so this treatment is good for any vata disorders that cause you to feel scattered and unable to focus. The herbs used in this treatment can improve cognitive function. It invigorates prana, making people feel energized and focused, especially those with a vata constitution. In this case, we use medicated ghee that has been infused with ashwagandha or with fresh juices such as gotukola. The gotukola leaves are from the Brahmi family, which has a number of strong health benefits. Ghee infused with Shatavari, which relieves stress and improves cognitive function.

SHAMANA NASYA (PALLIATIVE)

This is another nutritive treatment that calms the nervous system. It is especially indicated for those who can't stop the swirl of thoughts, for those who are workaholics, and people suffering from insomnia. The herbs commonly use include calamus to improve lucidity and Jatamansi, which promotes relaxation.

Some Nasya treatments that don't involve oil at all. Sometimes we use crushed powders, or even black pepper powder. The patient uses a straw to inhale this powder into the nose. This causes sneezing, which also clears the passages, opens the channels and increases prana in the head and neck. This is especially good for kapha types and those who suffer from stress. It opens up the deep channels and deep tissues and clears the nasal passages. If you suffer from frequent bouts of congestion when you wake up in the morning, or have a heavy, headachy feeling on most mornings, you might benefit from this dry Nasya. In fact, this is a type of Nasya that you have probably done accidentally at home. A little whiff of pepper powder will induce some sneezing. While you may not have noticed at the time, you probably felt lighter and clearer after you sneeze.

Preparing for Nasya

This is one technique in which you will need localized external oleation and heat to prepare the head and neck for the healing benefits of the herbs and oils. You will enjoy a vigorous massage of the face and neck. Your practitioner will massage and stimulate the sinus areas around your eyes. Remember that the face contains many marma points. These are vital energy centers that enable the flow of energy throughout the body. You utilize these centers whenever you laugh or frown and they can get blocked if underused or overused. The massage helps to activate these marma points and release the energy they hold so that the treatment can penetrate deeper into the sinuses.

Then your practitioner will wrap a hot pack in a warm, damp cloth and gently place this over your eyes, sinuses and neck. As an alternative, your practitioner may have you breathe in steam that has been infused with eucalyptus oil or clove drops. The warmth or steam stimulates and opens the nasal passages and sinuses so that they are ready to receive herbal infusions.

How Nasya is Administered

You will lie on a table with your head tilted slightly back so that the nostrils are facing upward. The practitioner will add a few drops of oil to each nostril. You may be asked to inhale sharply to draw the oils further into the nasal passages. Then you relax and let the oil do its work, while you receive more massage to the cheeks and forehead.

After some time, you can blow your nose to remove excess oil and any toxins.

Sometimes, the oil will contain a little bit of black pepper to stimulate the release of mucus. If you do get a little congestion in your throat, you may be given warm water with turmeric, salt and honey as a gargle to further cleanse and nourish the mouth and throat. One patient told us this treatment alone saved him from getting tonsillitis surgery. The procedure opened the channels of his throat and esophagus. Over time, it reduced the inflammation of his tonsils which meant that his doctor told him he no longer needed surgery.

In some cases, you might feel a burning sensation in the nose during Nasya. If this happens, your practitioner might add a couple of drops of ghee to calm down the tissues.

Powder Nasya. For this, your practitioner will ask you to inhale a pinch of powder. This may cause you to sneeze, but that is expected. An alternative is that you inhale powder that has been placed in a metal or paper tube. These powders are more cleansing than the oil based Nasya treatments. Common choices are ginger powder that is both warming and heating. Ginger tends to trigger sneezing that will clear the sinuses. Calamus powder is more nurturing, and can have a calming effect on vata disorders including anxiety while also sharpening memory and the senses.

Vapor/Steam Nasya. Leaves or other herbs are put into a pot of boiling water. You will cover your head with a towel and lean over the pot to inhale the steam. Common choices include lemongrass oil, which has a calming effect on the nervous system and a cooling effect on the body. Mint or Eucalyptus leaves help to open the nasal passages and release mucus. Any one of these choices will offer gentle decongestion without drying the tissues. This type of Nasya is safe and effective for anyone, including children and the elderly.

Results of Nasya

After the treatment, your practitioner will apply a warm cloth to your face and neck while you relax. Your sinuses may continue to water or produce mucus. There's no cause for alarm if this happens because the sinuses and throat are still rendering toxins. Your eyes may water a little bit, too. Afterward, you will be able to wash your face and neck and you may be encouraged to gargle with warm water to clear your throat. At this point, you will feel a complete lightness in your senses and in your mind. Some people say that the mood is almost like the high they experience after intense exercise. That makes sense because this improves the prana, or life energy, in the upper body and brain. Suddenly, everything seems clear. Everything seems possible.

My patients who suffer from seasonal depression say that this treatment works wonders for them in the winter. Many people exercise less in the winter causing their brains to release less dopamine and serotonin, which brings down their mood. The lack of exercise means that they aren't taking deep breaths to clear the channels of the respiratory system. They sit at a desk all day, and go to work when it's dark and come home when it's dark. Soon, they feel depressed and unable to concentrate. But if they schedule their panchakarma treatments in the late fall, they can get a Nasya treatment after which all the channels open again, and they feel light and sharp throughout the colder months and ready to tackle new challenges.

This is also one of the few treatments from which young patients can benefit. I have one patient who is just 11-years-old. He has muscular dystrophy. His condition doesn't just weaken his muscles. It also affects his cognitive function, his speech and his eyesight. And yet he has such a beautiful heart. He writes poems that he posts on his blog, and he has many friends at school. I've been working with him for several months, and have helped his parents start a routine at home before bedtime. They massage oil into his arms and legs, which nourishes the tissues and skin. Then they put drops of oil into his nose using a special ghee infused with special herbs. They do this without fail, and they notice that he sleeps better at night. He wakes refreshed and relaxed. It's no easy thing to go to school every day when you have significant physical and sensory challenges and his parents told me that many times he would face the day with apprehension instead of joy. But now he wakes and is excited to go to school. He feels that his senses are sharper and that he can more easily express himself. He is calm and alert.

Anyone can benefit from this same clarity. We have noticed that children as well as people with Vata imbalances benefit the most from such care.

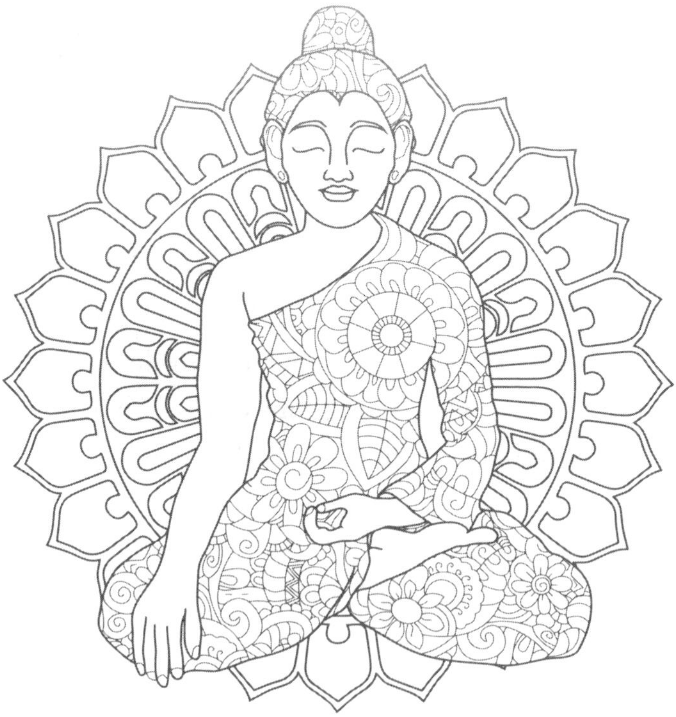

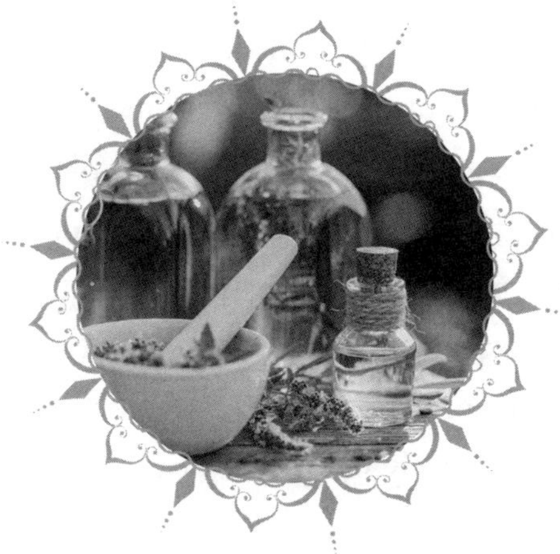

CHAPTER NINE

VIRECHANA

In this treatment, your practitioner will give you herbs or oils designed to push toxins out of the small intestines. This has the secondary benefit of cleansing the liver and gall bladder. Helps remove wastes and toxicity that would otherwise be absorbed into the blood.

It's used during panchakarma treatments because the poorvakarma has already loosened toxins from the tissues throughout the body and delivered them back into the digestive tract. You now need to flush those toxins out of the body before they can be reabsorbed.

You've probably already done a form of Virechana in your preparation for panchakarma. If you were directed to take a dose of castor oil, you were doing a pre-cleansing action to remove the ama stored in your small intestines. During a panchakarma, we are building on this process and this time removing the toxins recently loosened from your body's tissues. This is one of the few procedures that your practitioner may encourage you to do at home. Many people do some form of Virechana four times a year, on each solstice and equinox. As these seasonal changes happen, your doshas can use a little help staying in balance.

When some patients have an urgent need to balance pitta, they can require Virechana outside of a panchakarma regimen. Pitta disorders can come on suddenly in the summer months when pitta is dominant, but they can occur for other reasons as well.

A few months ago, a patient contacted me after his mother passed away. She had been sick for several years and this man had been her youngest son and the one who was closest to her. When she died, he immediately experienced a severe rash on his back. The skin was suddenly very inflamed, which coincided with his intense grief. In this case, with a sudden onset of pitta imbalance, a Virechana treatment can be very effective. I gave him some castor oil along with several herbs including magnesium, Brahmi, and Ashwagandha. He took the castor oil the next morning, which caused his small intestines to void and push the excess heat out of his body. The following morning the rash had decreased by about 50%. So, we did an additional cleanse the next week. After that, the rash had almost completely vanished. He agreed to do a final cleanse. And it cleared up completely! What we have to remember is that the skin is tied directly to our internal organs, and specifically the small intestine. We have to think of the skin as an emotional membrane around the body. Once this cleared up, he didn't need to do another Virechana treatment. This is not something you would do weekly or too often. It has to be done in response to what the body is telling you that it needs.

Who Benefits from Virechana

Anyone with a pitta-related imbalance can benefit from this treatment. We think of pitta imbalances as coming on in the summer when pitta is dominant. This is when people have migraines or chronic headaches, heartburn, and ulcers. Most skin conditions, including psoriasis, dermatitis, and eczema respond to this treatment. And some systemic conditions such as allergies. But this imbalance may come on any time with people of a pitta constitution. Anything to do with intestinal disorders, such as colitis or irritable bowel syndrome, liver problems, gallstones. These disorders resolve quickly with Virechana, particularly when people follow the appropriate lifestyle changes after the panchakarma.

This treatment has a cleansing effect on the stomach, kidneys, small intestine, the sweat glands, the liver, spleen and gall bladder.

It can have a powerful systemic effect on the body and can create emotional as well as physical healing. About a year ago, a young woman came to my clinic suffering from a terrible psoriatic arthritis rash that covered much of her body. She had been prescribed a steroid to control the rash, but it made her puffy and even more aggravated. Once we had a chance to talk more, I found that she was also suffering from insomnia because the rash was keeping her awake. And it was affecting her body image. She had lost contact with most of her friends. Upon further investigation, she had a lot of anger toward her parents, who had divorced when she was very young and who had both remarried. She had been raised in two households and felt torn between the two. This young woman was only 19-years-old. She had a serious pitta aggravation especially during the pitta time of life. Because this aggravation had gone on for so long, the disease process had already set in. She had started drinking as a young teenager and used that as a coping mechanism. I had to explain to her that alcohol is like throwing gasoline on a fire if the primary problem is pitta aggravation and inflammation.

I talked to her very seriously about how to change the course of her health and about letting go of some of this anger. I gave her a skin tonic to use. She agreed to a diet that would help cool the body and subdue the pitta energies. With a good diet in place and a regular exercise routine of yoga in the morning and evening, she was ready to prepare for the panchakarma treatment. I saw her every 15 days to check in on her diet and internal oleation. Within a month, her skin had started to clear up to the point where she could sleep through the night. She was ready for a full 7-day treatment. It's common for a pitta dominant person to need cooling agents during the poorvakarma. We sometimes use different oils such as sandalwood, or oils that contain mint, which also has a cooling effect. We might use oils infused with neem or aloe vera, both of which have a healing effect on the skin and help purify the blood. We still use steam heat to help pull out the toxins, but having cooling herbs and oils on the body helps prevent the body from creating more inflammation.

She struggled at first with the Virechana, because the viscous castor oil made her gag. But, her skin got about 10% better during the actual treatment. Skin conditions are very difficult to treat because everything you see on the surface of the skin correlates to other systemic problems in the body. Skin problems can often lurk under the surface if you aren't treating the whole body.

During the treatment, she kept a journal and we asked her to write down some of her grievances, the things that made her angry. This had the effect of processing the anger, getting it out of the head where it would circulate endlessly and instead put it down on paper. She also journaled about her body image and her goals for herself. What were her unique talents? We asked her what she wanted to accomplish with her life.

I continued to see her once a month after this treatment and her skin cleared up beautifully. She enrolled in college where she began to make career goals for herself. And when she saw me most recently, she said she sometimes looks back on those journal entries she made during her treatment and thinks she doesn't even recognize that person. She feels completely reborn.

How to Prepare for Virechana

All of the internal oleation that you have done before the pancha-karma and during the poorvakarma have prepared your body for this treatment. Typically, you will have three days of taking medicated ghee or other oily substance along with sweating to prepare the body. Your practitioner will probably have given you doses of what's known as bitter ghee, in which the ghee has been infused with dozens of healing herbs. This ghee helps to soften the tissues along the digestive tract and allow the herbs to absorb into your system and dislodge toxins.

You will be encouraged to eat about two and a half hours before the Virechana begins. And this meal will have a pitta quality. It might contain foods that are spicy, hot or sour. You have to wait the full two and a half hours after your meal to take the purgative substance because you don't want the food to still be digesting in the stomach. This will make the treatment less effective. After you eat, you will be discouraged from doing anything too taxing mentally or physically. Exercise, for example, will pull blood away from the digestive tract and into your muscles. If this happens, there is a chance that the toxins will also flow back into the tissues.

How Virechana is Administered

The type of substances given to you by your practitioner will depend on your body type. People with a pitta type body who typically have frequent bowel movements might be given a milder laxative. Those with a kapha constitution whose digestive tract may move more slowly will need a stronger laxative. Vata types often experience constipation and may need something that has an unctuous quality such as castor oil to move the ama out of the small intestine. Sometimes these substances are infused with medicinal herbs.

This is typically administered during the pitta time of day between 10 a.m. and 2 p.m. or in the evening before bed so that the laxative can work overnight. You will need to refrain from eating during this time. Some people do experience some cramping, but this feeling should pass as you rid the body of the stored ama. You should expect that in a couple of hours you will feel the urge to use the bathroom. A successful treatment usually produces between 4 and 6 stools, which will be solid at first, then liquid. Be sure to sip water after each bowel movement. You want to keep yourself hydrated. Your practitioner might give you some water that contains electrolytes if you are feeling dehydrated.

You will be asked to keep track of your bowel movements, the number, quality and consistency. And you will be asked how you feel after the procedure. In rare cases, the treatment fails to evacuate the bowels completely. If you take a laxative and nothing happens or there is only one bowel movement, and you feel bloated afterward, your practitioner may start the process again. This will mean taking more oil internally and sweating so the body can prepare for another dose. Once you've started the process of panchakarma and moved the toxins from the tissues and into the colon, it's important to get them out of the body entirely.

After Virechana, most people feel light, clear-headed and relaxed. Your practitioner will warn against vigorous exercise. It's important to rest and relax afterward. You will need a special diet in the days following Virechana. You should also avoid cold baths or iced beverages. The tissues along your digestive tract have been doing a lot of work and they need rest and warmth. This is a good time to sip teas and do a little journaling.

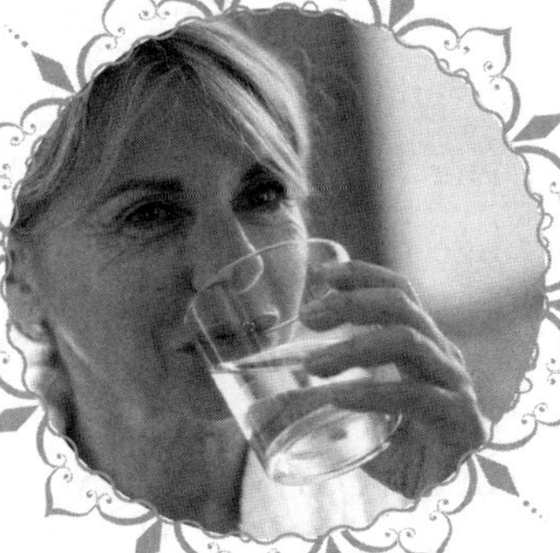

CHAPTER TEN

VAMANA & RAKTAMOKSHANA

There are two procedures that are part of traditional panchakarma that are rarely done in U.S. clinics because of legal issues. The first of these is Vamana, which is induced emesis or vomiting. The second is called Raktamokshana, which is a form of bloodletting. In India, practitioners may use a syringe to remove a small amount of blood from the patient (phlebotomy), or they may use leeches to draw blood from the body. Although you'll never encounter either of these procedures in a clinic that operates in the U.S., you might want to know that they exist and understand why a traditional panchakarma treatment in other countries might include these treatments.

Vamana

Most people associate vomiting with the flu or food poisoning, and therefore think of it as something uncomfortable and upsetting. Actually, regurgitation is a natural response to clearing the contents of the stomach if they seem to contain contaminants. This is also a quick way to remove irritants or mucus. If you have a pet, either a dog or cat, you are probably familiar with the way these animals induce vomiting in order to purge their stomachs. They don't do it because they have a virus or feel sick, but rather to cleanse the stomach and upper gastrointestinal tract. Dogs frequently eat grass in the spring, even though this will make them throw up. Many animals undertake something similar in the spring season as a way of clearing the body before a more active season.

It's true that humans have no such instinct for seasonal emesis. It's also true that purging can become a pathological response to emotional distress in some people. Vomiting should not be induced on a regular basis because it's not healthy. Taking laxatives regularly is also unhealthy. These tools should only be used under the guidance of a trained practitioner in order to restore the body to its natural balance and optimum functioning.

In India, where Ayurveda is practiced widely, many people engage in a form of Vamana according to their doctor's prescriptions. This is particularly true in the early spring. During winter, the sinuses, lungs and nasal passages get dry and irritated. Then when the spring comes and the rains start, everybody gets sick or congested. And these spring conditions are often further exacerbated by the rising pollen levels that can cause even more irritation. Those who suffer from seasonal allergies, spring colds, asthma, chronic congestion or headaches want to use Vamana to clear their systems in the early spring. In fact, there are so many people seeking this spring treatment that you can often find vomiting camps out in the open near Ayurvedic clinics. People know that in the springtime, it's time for a cleanse. You see people lined up in rows of chairs, sometimes 20 people to a row. And they all have a bucket. They are sitting and chatting with each other while someone goes from seat to seat handing out an herbal concoction that everybody drinks. And they gently regurgitate and leave.

There is another tradition among yogis called kunjal kriya, and this is a form of vomiting to cleanse the stomach and upper digestive tract. It involves ingesting about a gallon of warm saline water on an empty stomach, ideally first thing in the morning. Sometimes the saline water itself causes the body to expel the water. Sometimes the yogi needs to tickle the back of his throat. This is not done daily, but at various times to keep the digestion clean. It is considered to be one of the six cleansing actions used to maintain the body. You should know that this kunjal kryia works best for people who have had very pure diets for many years and who have very little deep-seated ama. If you are getting a panchakarma, you probably have ama that has already migrated away from the gut and this type of technique will not be effective.

Who Can Benefit from Vamana

If you travel to another country to get panchakarma, you might be prescribed Vamana if you have any of the classical kapha disorders. These include seasonal allergies, chronic congestion, headaches, or lethargy. Any disorder pertaining to the lungs might make you a candidate for this procedure. It's useful for some skin disorders, and obesity. It's also good for those who are holding onto negative emotions from the past. These can include prolonged grief, old resentments or long standing depression. These are the emotional signs of aggravated kapha.

How Vamana is Performed

Vamana is normally the first purification therapy done after several days of poorvakarma. It is usually done in the morning, during the kapha period of the day, meaning between 6 a.m. and 10 a.m. The night before, patients are encouraged to eat kapha aggravating foods, including dairy products, bananas, and black lentils. They are also told to get a good night's sleep. In the morning, you eat nothing, except perhaps some herbal tea.

For the procedure itself, patients are given between 4 and 8 cups of licorice tea. Then they ingest special herbs that are known to induce vomiting. Because of the liquid tea already in the stomach, the herbs can take up to 45 minutes to work. Patients will be told not to resist the urge to vomit, but to let it happen like a wave overtaking the body. The act itself should bring minimum discomfort, and a practitioner will be nearby to rub your back or hold your head if needed. This practitioner will also be taking your pulse and talking you through the process. If the urge to vomit never comes, the patient may be given additional licorice tea or encouraged to stimulate the back of the throat a little. But this is usually not necessary.

The signs that the treatment was successful include a feeling of lightness in the body, and an energetic mind. People usually feel a pleasant sense of hunger afterward, without feeling a strong urge to eat, which is also a good sign that the treatment was successful.

Afterward, patients are discouraged from eating or drinking anything for two to four hours in order to let the digestive tract settle down. After four hours, you can take some herbal tea and prepare for a light evening meal of soup or khichadi.

Raktamokshana

This treatment involves removing blood from the patient and it's the only other panchakarma procedure not offered in the US, because this type of procedure must be done by a licensed physician or phlebotomist. Yet, bloodletting has a long history inside Ayurveda as a means of purifying the blood. Sushruta, one of the most renowned Ayurvedic physicians in history, talked extensively about the blood as a main driver of human health. In fact, he thought of the blood as the fourth dosha. He was so influential that when the ancient Greeks adopted and adapted Ayurvedic principles, they turned the three doshas into the four humors. The Greeks considered blood to be the fourth—and most dominant—humor. It's the blood that nourishes the tissues. When the body's pitta energy is aggravated, the blood becomes heated and moves to the periphery of the body where it creates skin disorders. If you get panchakarma treatment in another country and you suffer from chronically irritated skin, systemic inflammation or blood disorders of any kind, you can expect the practitioner to consider Raktamokshana as a possible treatment. The thinking is that removing a small amount of blood helps the body rebalance pitta and resolve these disorders.

How Raktamokshana is Performed

There are many ways to safely remove blood from the body, but Raktamokshana usually involves just two methods. The first is through a syringe, and the second is with leeches. Each procedure is done after the oil massage and sweating to prepare the body, and each time the patient will likely be put on a liquid diet in the hours beforehand.

SIRAVYADHA

This is done with a syringe and it works pretty much the way you would have blood drawn for a medical test. The area around the blood draw will be thoroughly cleaned and then the practitioner would put pressure on the vein to make it stand out. While most people give blood from a vein on the inside of the arm, in Raktamokshana any number of veins could be used. Sometimes the blood is drawn from near the area where the patient is experiencing symptoms. The amount of blood drawn varies according to the diagnosis of the patient, but it's usually between 60 and 80 ccs of fluid, or about 2 ounces. After removing the needle, the practitioner will apply pressure along with astringent fluids or herbs such as turmeric and licorice to close the tiny wound.

In the old days, a practitioner would have made a small puncture in the vein to allow the blood to flow. This is similar to the way western doctors used to conduct bloodletting in the 16th and 17th centuries before the practice fell out of fashion. After letting the blood flow freely for a couple of minutes, the doctor would apply an astringent powder to close the wound.

JALAUKA

This is a Sanskrit word that means leeches. The procedure is actually quite safe and painless. More researchers are becoming interested in leech therapy to reduce inflammation and to help in wound healing. It has been used successfully to dissolve blood clots and to relieve precursory symptoms of osteoarthritis. Leeches are frequently used in recovery from cosmetic and reconstructive surgery. Leech saliva contains anticancer properties, but researchers are still exploring this phenomenon.

In India, Ayurvedic physicians keep leeches in plain water where they are fed and tended to with great care. Then before the procedure, the leeches would be smeared with a paste containing turmeric and mustard that will act as a disinfectant and increase the ability of the leech to do its work. There are many techniques for choosing the spot at which the leach should attach. Once it is attached, the practitioner will cover it with damp gauze to keep it moist. Patients are asked to report any itching or discomfort during the procedure because there should be no pain. Itchiness is a sign that the leech has drawn enough blood and needs to be removed. Usually, they disengage on their own and don't need to be coaxed. In most cases, practitioners use between three and six leeches on one patient, each of which draws out a small amount of blood. Once the treatment ends, any small wound on the skin would be treated with astringents and herbs. The leeches are then put in a water tank that contains turmeric or salt, which causes the leeches to regurgitate the blood. And then they are moved to a clean tank. Leeches are not to be used again, not even on the same patient, for at least 15 days.

Regardless of which type of bloodletting is done, the patient needs rest afterward. Patients should be told to avoid excess cold and heat or exertion through exercise. They will also be given a diet that's beneficial for the blood, including a warm food that contain ghee.

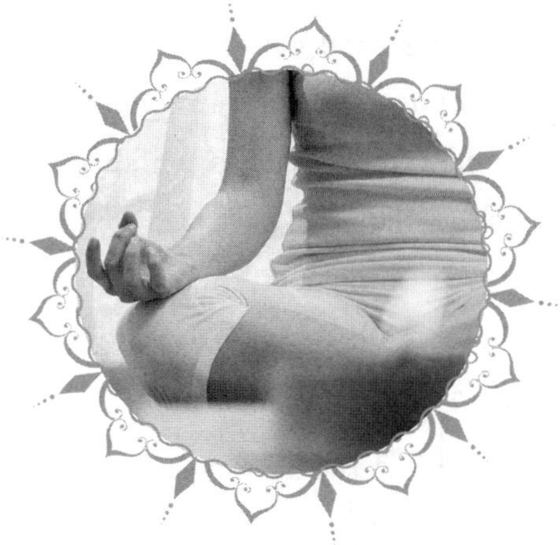

CHAPTER ELEVEN

THE EMOTIONAL CLEANSE

There is no predicting what can happen during a series of treatments. Many people feel deep relaxation. Some can even go through a kind of transcendent experience, one in which they feel connected to their life's purpose or the planet as a whole. For others, the experience has its ups and downs. On some days, the massage or steam feels relaxing, while on others it feels a little intrusive or uncomfortable, or even boring. Everyone gets a little bit concerned before their first basti. It is an odd sensation, but most people get used to it and enjoy the light and cleansed feeling afterward.

For most of our patients, the treatments offer a pampering that is alien to them. They haven't been nourished and cared for in this way since they were babies. Or it hasn't happened at all. As a result, the treatments cause them to feel physically safe and happy in a way they can't remember experiencing before.

In addition to the physical sensations of treatment that trigger an emotional response, you will be aware of old feelings and sensations as well. The treatments are unblocking emotional experiences from years or even decades earlier. The body often stores old traumas and stressors. It even encases them in fat. The scrubbing, steaming and oil treatments release these blockages and the toxins flow into the digestive tract or to the skin, where they can be eliminated. And this isn't always pleasant. You may feel anger or sadness or have memories resurface of things you've forgotten about.

The Three Bodies

When we speak of detoxifying, we usually mean the physical body.

But there are many emotional and even spiritual benefits of panchakarma that go beyond physical purification. Ayurveda recognizes that the mind, the body and the spirit are woven together. Any impurities stored in the body affect the mind. Any emotional disturbances also disrupt the body's function. And any treatment that acts upon the body to dislodge old toxins and remove them will also have a similar effect on your emotional health. Health and disease can have two locations, the body and the mind.

THE BODY HAS THREE LAYERS

THE PHYSICAL BODY

This is sometimes referred to as the gross body, but it is the physical manifestation of any person. It contains all the tissues, organs and processes that keep the body alive and functioning. This is where the panchakarma interacts with you most directly.

THE CAUSAL BODY

This is sometimes described as the seed or origin of any individual, and it consists of a field of potential. When we cleanse the physical body, we remove the artificial veil between your conscious state and the deep potential in you.

THE SUBTLE BODY

This is a layer of experience and emotion that exists between the other two bodies. The subtle body can contain the emotions, experiences, feelings, and particularly those that are stuck. These include psycho-emotional toxins that have been stuck. The memories of past injuries and traumas beyond the physical level. When you detox the physical body, you are opening the channels of the subtle body as well.

The process of panchakarma often allows you to access impulses and insights that have been hidden from you. I've had patients go through panchakarma and realize that they want to change professions or end a relationship or move to a different country. I always urge people to receive these insights with gratitude but to hold off on acting out any drastic changes. Sometimes the feelings you have during treatment will continue to evolve after treatment ends. A few times, patients have had only a glimmer of understanding about how they've lived their lives and these feelings grow as they get home and the treatment continues to work.

I recently saw a woman who runs a highly successful business. She built the business when she was a young single mother. She is now nearly 70 years old and her children have children of their own. She resisted coming to panchakarma even though she was struggling with a number of health issues. I kept hearing the same excuse, that she was too busy to take time off. At one point I asked her bluntly whether her dozens of employees ever take vacation. Of course, she said yes. And then I asked why she wasn't allowed to take a vacation for self-care, even if it would improve her health. Finally, she relented. During treatment, the only thing she wanted to talk about or journal about was her business and what it meant to her. On the very first day of treatment, I asked her what would be left of her life if the business suddenly disappeared. What would her life look like? I asked her to journal about this. She went through seven days of treatment and she journaled every day. She told me that she has no friends, no relationships. She rarely sees her grandchildren and never does anything for fun. Her work day starts at 6 a.m. and she is frequently the last person to leave the office.

Over the course of the seven days, I watched her body soften. She lost weight, but more importantly, she lost all of the tension that had been haunting her. We talked about some of the things she might like to have in her life in addition to the business. She brainstormed ways to limit her work life and to re-connect with old friends. She also realized that she had been clinging to the business and to the idea of working constantly because the business had become her entire identity. When she was young, she liked the idea of building a brand and being the face of that brand because he boosted her confidence. Now, she wasn't so sure. Now, it seemed more like a crutch.

That was two years ago. She has come back for panchakarma every year since that first year and has recently told me that during that first treatment, she had an idea about what it would be like to retire and give up the business entirely. She didn't do it right away. Gradually, the idea began to grow inside her mind. Over the course of the next year, it kept nagging at her. She was finally in touch with what she needed instead of what she thought she needed. This past winter, she told me that she has a plan in place to turn the business over to her children and spend some time enjoying her life on her own terms. This is the goal of panchakarma.

How Body Type Affects Your Response

Everyone responds differently to a course of treatment. But your body type may predict how the emotional healing may manifest.

| VATA |

Those with a vata body type usually respond best to treatments with oil. They often experience dry skin, constipation and variable appetite. When depleted, they are often scattered or anxious. For them, the oil treatments are a kind of balm on the entire system because the vata tissues are often starved of proper fats. When those of a vata constitution have dry tissues, they experience creaky joints and the ama sticks to their digestive tract much more readily.

I remember one patient coming for treatment who was terribly anxious in her life. She was anxious all day at work, even though her work was going well and then she would go home at night and be overcome with depression. She told me she would often cry late into the night. She didn't know why. After some consultations, she confessed that she was unhappy in her career, that she was afraid that she would never find a relationship. Truthfully, she didn't like her life and didn't know what steps to take to change it.

Normally, I would counsel someone like this to get on the right nutritional path, get a good healthy schedule in place with some exercise, a better sleep routine and some journaling, and let the body balance itself over time. But her level of anxiety during the day and the depression at night worried me, and so I encouraged her to also try a panchakarma.

Vata types love the oil, the heat. They find it relaxing and nourishing. In Sanskrit, the word Sneha can mean oil but it also means to bind and to love. The oil massage offers nourishment to the skin and the mind. For vata types, it can be transformative on its own.

On the first day, my patient had the oil massage and heat, then we poured oil over her head. Then she had a basti. Her body absorbed every drop of oil we used. And afterward, she looked and felt completely different. She looked several years younger. She stayed for seven days and told me that she could feel her body changing on a cellular level. She journaled about her goals and even made sketches of the type of person she would like to meet. When your body is detoxing, it is also releasing old feelings. In her case, it liberated the feeling that she didn't deserve love. Within a couple of months, she told me that she had found a partner who looked very similar to her sketches.

PITTA

My pitta patients are often bringing the same drive and ambition to the clinic that they use in their regular lives. They do best when we help them slow down and relax. One of my patients was a life coach for CEOs. He was used to giving people advice that they resisted, and he liked battling with these people, trying to charm them into doing what he thought they needed to do to reach their goals. He was busy and had gained a reputation as someone who could be tough on his clients.

I told him that during his panchakarma he was to engage in five days of silence. No TV, no computer, no texts. The whole staff would know about this silent retreat and honor it. I gave him some books to read with certain passages marked. His routine would be to come to the clinic to do some stretching, then meditate and sit in silence for three hours. Then he would have the oil massage and heat. I told him to leave the oil on his body for another two or three hours. Then he could go back to his room to take a long bath. He could take a walk in the woods for exercise, then eat a light dinner of soup and go to bed. He had a very simple routine to keep and he struggled with it at first. He didn't know how to be alone with his own thoughts. I sometimes joke to my patients, saying. "It's a panchakarma because I'm going to punch the karma out of you." Sometimes it does work like that. We are turning the body inside out every day. Through this process you can have the distance to see yourself and your life objectively. You see who you are.

After five days we started talking for the last two days. He said he felt completely quiet, centered, and relaxed. One insight was that he should change the nature of his work. He felt that he wasn't seeing his clients fully. He was just telling them what he thought was right. He wasn't listening to them, and he'd never helped them see their own skill set. Instead he just dazzled everybody with his sales pitch, but nobody knew who he was. He decided to change his entire approach to consulting and he told me that he never would have understood his own behavior without this silent retreat.

KAPHA

People with a kapha constitution often come to the clinic for weight loss issues. But emotionally, they are also often hanging on to some trauma from the past. One of my kapha clients was a young bank manager. She was carrying about 100 extra pounds and she told me that she had become very self-conscious about her body. She had come to the point where she was using her sick days to avoid going to work where she had to greet people and talk to people. As we talked, she said that she didn't like herself at all. She was very depressed. She went on the pre panchakarma diet for a month. During that time, she lost 11 pounds. She came to the clinic for seven days of treatment. She was given a strong basti and we used dry scrubs to circulate the lymph system. She kept a journal and answered questions I gave her about how she felt about herself. What emerged was an understanding that she had become sexually active as a young teenager and had been in some abusive relationships. Afterward, she grappled with the desire to be invisible to others. This was what precipitated her weight gain throughout high school and college.

On about the fourth day, I saw the change in her. She began to think about herself differently and was able to let go of some of the trauma. I had always known that she had great intelligence and had been selling herself short in her job and in her life. But on that fourth day, she began to see all of this, too. She could finally take her thoughts out of the past and focus more directly on her future. We talked about her goals. How should her career unfold? What kind of relationship would she want?

She told me that she'd always felt as though there was a heavy, wet blanket around her body and a dense cloud of fog in her mind. Now, it was falling away. She felt more alive, clearer in body and mind. We kept her on a program of good diet and self-care and I still hear from her sometimes. She has lost more than 60 pounds and is taking some banking exams and more responsibility at work.

This is what I mean when I say there are issues in your tissues. The toxins in your body are changing your biochemistry and giving you false signals. Once we clean out the cells, you can let go of old trauma and focus on what you want in life.

The Healing Crisis

Not every emotional transformation comes easily, though. Each day of a panchakarma reaches deeper into the tissues and this can flush out old and uncomfortable debris. After a couple of days people begin to be more emotional. Maybe they feel like crying or they fell a long forgotten rage. Sometimes they feel light and elated also for no real reason. And the body is reacting, too. There are certain types of emotional and physical response to the treatments. And you should be aware of these so that you don't become alarmed during the process.

| FATIGUE |

People sometimes say they are so tired that they feel like they've got the flu. They get sleepy in the early evening and may sleep for 12 hours at a time. It's as though they finally feel how run down the body has become. Remember that your body is working hard to give up these toxins. It needs plenty of rest. Of course, some people have the opposite problem. They sleep during all the treatments and then don't feel tired at night.

| HIGH ENERGY |

After the first wave of exhaustion, you might feel the energy rebound. We have people who start to feel so good that they want to go out and run ten miles or hike a mountain. They get very ambitious and we have to insist that they take it easy instead. In a few cases, people have reported changes in their sexual appetite. One man came to the clinic and he said he'd had no libido for many years, but then on the third or fourth day of treatment, he suddenly awakened to it again. The body really does reinvent itself.

CHANGES IN APPETITE

Some people don't feel like eating much during the treatment. Others have a ravenous appetite. I had one patient recently who was on a restricted diet of kichadi and leafy vegetables. But her Agni had become so strong that she was eating four times as much food as usual. You may also experience food cravings for things you know you shouldn't eat. Some people crave alcohol, even if they haven't had a drink in years. It's important to stick to the dietary restrictions during the treatments. And these cravings usually pass.

ACHES AND PAINS

Headaches are common in the first couple of days, as is some stiffness in the joints or body aches. The body may be throwing a fit as the toxins start to stream out. You may be conscious of old injuries and experience some discomfort in those areas. I've had people show me a swollen lymph node and ask if it's serious. This is actually a good sign that things are moving along properly. The body is actively working to rebalance itself.

SENSORY SENSITIVITY

People often find that their sense of smell sharpens in a way that's distracting. They may feel nausea after treatment, or waves of heat coming off the body. Or they have itchy skin. In a few cases, a rash will develop on the skin or an existing rash will flare up. You might have night sweats or the heart may start pounding in the night. Or they feel that they might be hallucinating in the night because their dreams are so vivid. This is all normal.

BODILY ODORS

This one should be obvious. Ama is foul smelling stuff and when it starts to come out your body's odor will change temporarily. People complain that their urine stinks, and that their bowel movements are gross. They have bad breath, and their sweat stinks. For me, this is just another day at the office. It's just a sign that things are working as they should.

WEIGHT LOSS

It's not uncommon to lose ten pounds in a seven-day panchakarma. One of my patients lost seven pounds in two days. It was mostly water weight. The truth is that once you wipe out the initial layer of toxins, the body begins to burn more fat. Most people don't complain about this side effect. And the weight loss continues after the treatment ends, especially if you eat carefully to avoid building up more ama.

It's difficult to predict how your body will react to the stress of panchakarma. Rest assured that any uncomfortable symptoms will pass and you will feel better. People can tend to have a bumpier ride if they have been on a lot of medications in the past. This includes chronic antibiotic use, which tends to dry the system and wipe out the gut flora. Fertility treatments also expose women to high doses of hormones that have a lasting effect. In these cases, you may need additional preparatory treatments such as enemas at home in the weeks before you go to the clinic.

People also struggle if they haven't prepared adequately by adhering to the preparatory diet. If you've had poor eating habits for many years, you may need to clean up your diet for more than one month. You may need several castor oil cleanses at home before you come in. Your practitioner can also modify your treatments if you are really struggling.

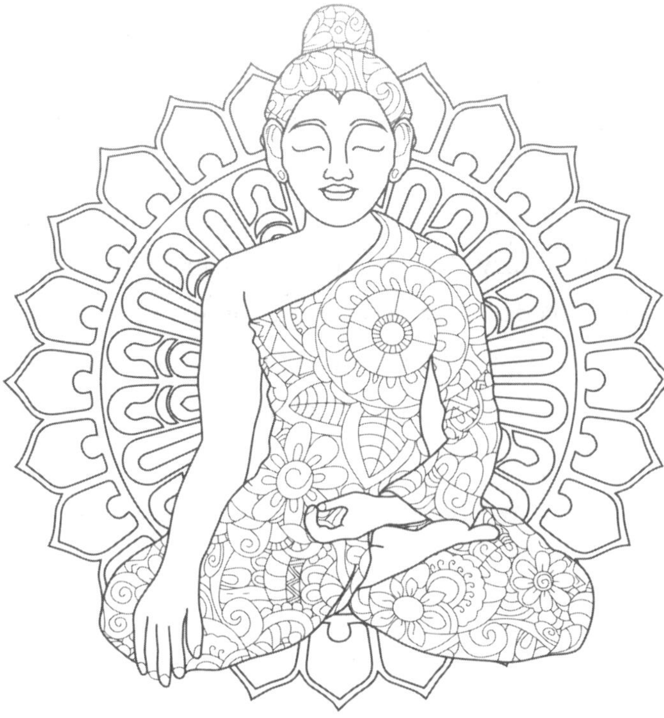

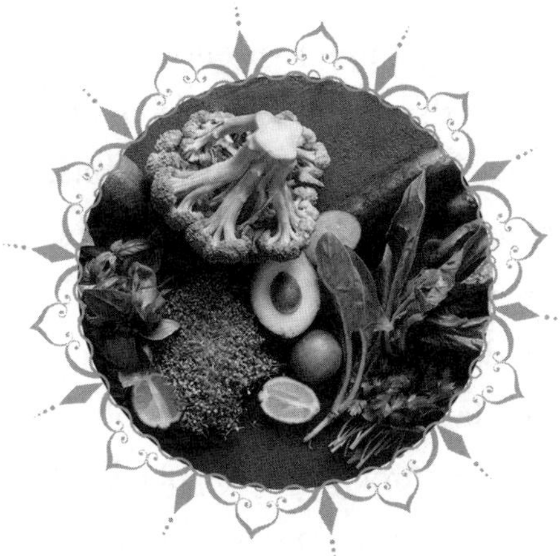

CHAPTER TWELVE

POST PANCHAKARMA

It may be tempting to think that once your visit to the clinic for daily treatments is over, that the whole healing process has been completed. This is not true. There are three critical phases to panchakarma and each one needs to be carried out faithfully. The first is preparation, which you did before you came to the clinic. You changed your diet and exercise routine and did some oleation on your own. Then the second phase was carried out in the clinic, when your body did the hard work of shedding excess toxins through treatments. The third phase is no less important, and that's what you do as you re-enter your life.

Panchakarma therapies go on for several days. Some people can do just three days of therapy, while others stay for a full seven days. In India, some patients remain at a clinic for two to three weeks to fully cleanse and heal. At some point, the therapies end for every patient, and it's time to prepare to re-enter your life. When your treatment ends, you will probably feel relaxed and balanced. You will likely have new insights about your life and relationships. At the same time, most people don't have much of an appetite, and they often feel sensitive to overstimulation. This is not the time to throw yourself back into work or crowded social settings or to celebrate your recovery by treating yourself to alcohol or junk food. Your body has been doing a lot of hard work ridding itself of ama and environmental toxins, and you want to treat yourself gently at first.

People often get excited by their higher levels of energy and the weight loss they experienced during treatment. But there may be other tangible benefits that you enjoy. One woman came in for a panchakarma even though she told me she didn't believe in detox or Ayurveda. But she had some kind of undiagnosed autoimmune problem. She was fatigued, sluggish and bloated. She had digestive problems. Her doctor suspected Lyme disease but couldn't diagnose it. A functional medicine expert suggested fibromyalgia. So she came in for a full seven days and left feeling great, better than she had in years. All of her symptoms were gone. Ten days after the treatment ended, she went in for an annual checkup and blood work only to discover that her cholesterol had dropped by 40 points. Her doctor was floored because he had begged her to go on statins and she'd always refused. Now she didn't need them. She had never dreamed that the treatment would do this much good for her. She's a believer now.

To prepare for this post panchakarma phase, you will meet with your practitioner to learn new habits that you will carry forward to protect your body from toxins in the future. This entails learning about:

DAILY ROUTINE	This includes setting a healthy schedule that includes exercise, meditation and five senses therapy that you can do on your own.
DIET	You will learn how to recharge your appetite in phases and how to eat to maintain your doshic balance in the weeks after therapy.
RASAYANA	These herbal supplements will protect your body's doshic balance and improve the flow of vital energy through the body.

The Daily Routine

Your practitioner will meet with you on the last day of panchakarma to explain your ideal daily routine in the first weeks after treatment. It's a little bit different for everyone, but most people will be advised to minimize electronic stimulation. So, you won't be diving into answering all of the emails you missed during treatment or binge-watching television shows the morning after your treatment. Instead, you will want to continue with meditation, journaling and quiet thoughts for the first couple of days. This is particularly true if you've had sweeping insights during treatment. Many times patients come to a new understanding of the choices they've made and announce that they are going to quit a job or sever a relationship that has been difficult. Resist the urge to do these things. Your insights will evolve over time, and this is not the time to charge into battle with yourself or your loved ones.

Good sleep supports the body, so you will be advised to get to bed early, no later than 10:30 and rise at the same time every day. At first, many patients say that they have so much energy that they fear they won't be able to sleep at night. But the body is naturally tired from treatment and if you avoid electronics in the evening, you will find that sleep comes naturally and you can reach a deep state of relaxation easily.

Light yoga in the morning and evening will also feel good and energizing in these first few days. Gradually, you can return to your normal levels of exercise. This is a good time to practice listening to your body and giving it what it needs.

Your practitioner may give you other specific guidelines based on your body type or the season in which you receive treatment. These may include specific foods or exercises to avoid.

It's important to follow these guidelines. You may feel wonderful and rejuvenated, and yet the body is in a little bit of a vulnerable state. The tissues will be working to rebuild and rebalance themselves and you need to be gentle with yourself. Putting too much stress on the body right away can have consequences. One of my patients left the clinic after her last day of treatment without telling me that she was scheduled to take a business trip overseas the next day. Instead of gently recovering, she instead boarded a crowded flight. She ate airplane food and drank wine and got very little sleep because she was staring at a computer screen furiously preparing for her meetings. By the time she landed, her headache was so intense that she couldn't function. That's when I got an emergency call from Hong Kong and prescribed a laxative to push out that newest wave of ama. It was not easy for her to find castor oil, but once she took this additional treatment she felt better and agreed to take it easy for the rest of the trip.

The Post Treatment Diet

Your digestive tract is the primary means for processing nourishment and eliminating toxins. For the duration of your treatment, your body has been focused on the second function. Toxins that had been residing in your tissues were pulled out and thrust into the throat, stomach and intestines. These tissues are pretty exhausted. In fact, you may have very little appetite, and that's okay. You can rebuild your appetite slowly in a process called the samsarjan krama, or the graduated diet. It will gently coax the body into taking nutrition again. Once your digestive tract awakens, you will feel more hungry and more energized by food. The trick is to take it easy at first. Remember that this phase should last an equal number of days as the panchakarma treatment itself. If you've had a seven-day treatment, then gradually reintroduce foods for an additional seven days.

PEYA	Your first meal after treatment should ideally be the kind of food you would give to a baby. I recommend cooking 1/3 cup of basmati rice in 4 cups of water for 25 minutes. It's likely that the result will be a thin gruel. If some grains of rice remain, you can strain them out and drink just the liquid.
VILEPI	For the next phase, you can cook the same amount of rice in 2 cups of water for 25 minutes. This will result in something more like a soup. You can eat both the rice grains and the water.
YUSHA	The next phase adds mung beans to your rice soup. Soak the beans for two hours prior to your meal, then cook them along with the rice.

After this phase, you can begin to add vegetables that have been steamed as well as ghee. This will more closely approximate the traditional dish of khichadi. You can then add nuts and spices.

Eventually, you will return to a normal diet that includes the various foods, including eggs, meat (if you eat meat) and a wide variety of vegetables. Your practitioner will probably caution you against eating certain foods based on your body type. Each person is different, and some people can't tolerate dairy without building up ama. Some people require a diet high in healthy fats, or certain spices, while others should use caution. Most people should avoid dull and heavy foods such as breads, sweets and simple carbs. Eating the foods right for your body and the season will help support your body as it continues to heal and gain energy.

Many patients notice that their taste buds have changed. Their food cravings remain, but these are illusory. They may take a bite of a piece of candy or junk food that they previously enjoyed and find that it tastes wrong or different. This is actually a good thing. It means that your body really has changed, and it craves a good, clean diet. One of my patients told me that he has trouble eating any of the foods he used to enjoy. Only now does he understand how over salted most snack foods are and how they don't taste like actual food. The desserts he used to crave now taste too sweet. His taste buds have become so sensitive that he revels in plainer fare. Sometimes patients call me to say that their cravings for bad food have continued and they feel that going through the panchakarma gives them a free pass to eat poorly because they have been so newly cleansed. I caution them to stay strong. You will continue to reap the benefits of the treatments for several months if you continue to eat a clean diet. This will help you maintain the strong energy levels you are feeling as you transition back into your daily activities.

Rasayana

Your practitioner will probably meet with you a week or so after the treatment has ended to do an additional evaluation and to talk about how you are feeling. At this time, you may be given special herbal supplements to keep you on track or to assist with any chronic conditions you may have. These are called Rasayana, or rejuvenation treatments. They are frequently herbal concentrates mixed with ghee, honey or jam. You won't be given these herbs until your digestive tract is up and running again. At this point, we can assume that your digestion is working at full speed and that your body's channels are open and clear. You will take a dose of these first thing in the morning when your stomach is empty.

These herbal preparations will be chosen based on your physical needs going forward. Some help with bones and joints, while others help with emotional stability or clarity in thinking. There are even special Rasayana preparations that help with insomnia.

I do caution people not to take other herbal supplements beyond the Rasayana treatments in the weeks after a panchakarma. Your body is highly sensitive to herbal remedies. Any dose will be twice as powerful now as it was before the treatment. Taking high doses of vitamins or even other Ayurvedic preparations may overwhelm the system. Many of my patients have been taking a daily Triphala or some ashwagandha powder for their own reasons before treatment. But in the weeks immediately following, you should leave those alone.

Using Panchakarma Treatments on Your Own

Many of my patients like to do a panchakarma treatment annually. They pick a time in the year when they might normally suffer from seasonal disorders, either allergies in the early summer or dryness and low-level depression in the winter, and just before that season starts, they come for a panchakarma and this gives them protection against the difficult season. It relieves the symptoms they might otherwise suffer during a difficult time of year because the doshas have been balanced.

A few of my patients have decided that they loved the panchakarma treatments so much that they want to come back the next month and do it all again. I urge people not to do this. According to Ayurveda, the best times to undergo panchakarma is during spring and fall. These seasons bring the most transitions to the body. For many people, this is a time when their bodies become susceptible to toxins or unhealthy habits. This is when minor doshic imbalances can become more extreme and disruptive. Colds, allergies and headaches are more common during these seasons. These conditions can be directly treated by panchakarma in the right season.

Even if you decide that you can only schedule a panchakarma once a year, you will reap tremendous rewards.

But I would urge people not to try to undergo this treatment more than twice a year. This is a comprehensive procedure and with too much repetition you risk wearing out your body. Think of your body as a complex cloth. A panchakarma treatment is like a putting the cloth in the laundry where it is scrubbed free of dirt. But if you wash the cloth over and over again, you eventually wear it down until it's threadbare. We don't want this.

If you do feel that you need a little tune up between treatments, you can do some of these individual actions on your own.

FIVE SENSES THERAPY

This is another name for panchakarma. During panchakarma the treatments address every one of the body's senses. You will receive drops for the ears, the eyes, the nose. These oil drops are tailored for your body's constitution and your specific health needs. Taken during treatment, they rejuvenate your senses. We often give patients oil preparations to use at home. Only the dosage is different. At the clinic, we use a higher dose as part of the healing therapy. At home, you will continue to use these drops at a smaller dose as part of your maintenance program. We call this a Five Senses Therapy Kit.

DAILY OIL MASSAGE

You can do your own version of the oil massages you received in the clinic. Simply heat up a little bit of sesame oil and rub it into your skin before stepping into a hot bath or shower. This does wonders for the mood, particularly if you often suffer from vata imbalances. Any time you are scattered, anxious or overwhelmed, you can use this self-massage to calm down and get grounded. This is particularly calming at the end of the day. Many of my patients consider this an indispensable part of their daily routine, especially in the winter when the air is so dry.

NASAL OIL DROPS

Anyone who suffers from snoring can benefit from this daily habit. Put some sesame oil into a little eyedropper and put a couple of drops in each nostril right before bed. Pinch the nose shut and inhale as you let go. Let the oil travel up and into the nose a little bit. It's okay if some of it trickles down your throat. This lubrication technique has cured many snorers among my patients and I've been told that it has saved more than one marriage.

EAR DROPS

You can also use sesame oil as drops in your ears. These drops help soften any ear wax and keep your ears from becoming clogged with wax. They are also useful when the air is dry during the winter, and when you are flying anywhere. Airplanes create a notoriously dry environment. The dehydration that your body suffers, even during a short flight, can disrupt your sleep and your mood for days afterward. A few drops in the ears will keep them moist and will help you relax.

EYE DROPS

Many people suffer from eye strain because we spend so much time staring at screens all day. Specially prepared eye drops contain herbal preparations in saline solution that can help relieve eye strain and redness. One or two drops per eye before bedtime will offer relief from tired eyes and headaches. They can also reduce the formation of cataracts and other debilitating eye conditions.

OIL PULLING

This treatment lubricates the gums and tissues inside your mouth. You simple put a little bit of oil in your mouth and swish it around for up to ten minutes. It could be almost any kind of edible oil, but many people use coconut oil. Don't worry about swishing it around vigorously, just let it move around your teeth and gums. This will clean out bad bacteria, nourish your gums and can resolve any issues with bad breath. Many people start their oil pulling before getting into the shower and then spit it out after the shower is over.

CASTOR OIL CLEANSE

You are already familiar with this cleanse as it was part of your panchakarma preparation. But it is also a powerful tool to use after your treatment ends. Your doctor will advise you on how often to repeat the cleanse in the months ahead. Your schedule will depend upon your body's constitution and your general health. Some people need to repeat the castor oil cleanse in as little as 15 days, while others will use it monthly or every three months.

Take a teaspoon of castor oil first thing in the morning on an empty stomach. If you can't stomach the taste, you can mix it with a little grapefruit juice and drink it quickly. Refrain from eating for most of the rest of the day until you have finished several bowel movements. In the evening, eat lightly and go to bed a little bit early. This is great for people who often have pitta imbalances such as skin rashes, acne, irritable bowels, or difficulties with anger or emotional irritation. Many people do this four times a year, once at each solstice and at each equinox. You can even do a castor oil cleanse every month, if it works well for you. I've often advised patients to do this monthly if they need extra help detoxing or resetting the digestive fire. If you are a woman, make sure to do the cleanse before your menstruation begins. This will help regulate your periods and alleviate PMS.

Processing Your Emotions

One of the greatest benefits of the panchakarma is its ability to eliminate emotional debris from past traumas. Most people experience great insights about how they want to live and how they relate to others after treatment. Some people announce on the third day of treatment that they want to quit their jobs or leave their spouse because they've realized that these situations are toxic. I encourage people to ride the wave of healing before they make such huge changes in their lives. Once the cleanse is complete and you have reintroduced your normal healthy diet, then is the time for action. You may find that you don't in fact want to change your whole life, but rather find that you want to behave differently in your life. This is a big enough change as it is.

A few of my patients have decided to make big changes after they got home and reacclimated. During the treatment, they gained insights about what they wanted to change and also about how to make these changes in a responsible way. This is an important distinction. You can't just go home and throw grenades around. You have to have a vision. In a good panchakarma treatment, your practitioner will be working with you on that vision of your new self. Make sure that your daily routine is sustainable and conducive to health and wellness.

One of my patients was a young woman living in a rural area and working in the family business. She felt that she was stuck in a small town doing a job she didn't like, but she didn't feel that she could leave without disappointing her parents. She was angry and frustrated, and unable to find a relationship. This anger and frustration was causing depression, insomnia and skin rashes. She came for a seven-day treatment during which we told her to observe total silence. Every day, we gave her a topic to journal about. One day she wrote about her parents. Another day, she wrote about her ideal job, or her ideal living situation. We asked her to envision the perfect life for herself, where she lived, what kind of friends and relationships she would have, how much money she would need in this new life. She did this as we were going through the different treatments to remove the physical toxins. At the end, she felt so empowered and so clear about what she wanted. She went home and coolly told her parents that she needed something different. And then she started looking for work online. A couple of months later, she wrote to me to say that she'd found a job and an apartment in a much larger community. She even sent me copies of her journal entries where she had envisioned this future and they matched perfectly with what she had found. There's something incredibly powerful in taking the time to relax and know what you want. But she would never have found all this clarity without first ridding herself of the old emotional toxins.

It may sound esoteric at times, but as you go into the depth of what you want, you can manifest many things. There are so many layers of separation and disconnection from your true self. And this is what panchakarma addresses.

Post Panchakarma Recipes

These are recipes that many of my patients have used in the days and weeks after a panchakarma. The first recipe is for Peya, the soupy rice mixture that you will consume for a few meals after the treatment ends. It will help fire up your digestion and prepare you for more complex meals.

| PEYA |

This is a kind of thin rice soup. In a saucepan, combine 2 quarts of water with 1 cup short grain basmati rice. Bring to a boil, cover and lower the heat to simmer for 20 minutes until the rice is very soft. Eat as a soup.

| VILEPI |

This is very similar to Peya, but it's a little bit thicker. You would use four parts of water for every one part of rice. Combine in a saucepan 4 cups of water and one cup of rice. Bring to a boil, then cover and reduce the heat to simmer for 20 minutes until the rice is tender.

For this soup, you can add a tablespoon of ghee and a pinch of spices, such as ginger, turmeric or coriander for taste.

| YUSH |

This simple soup contains yellow split mung beans, which are very easy to digest. Heat 4 cups of water to boiling and add one cup of basmati rice and ½ cup of mung beans. You can also add ½ teaspoon of salt a teaspoon of dried ginger powder or 1 teaspoon of freshly grated ginger and a pinch of ground black pepper. You can also add 1 tablespoon of ghee. Cover and reduce the heat to simmer for 15 minutes.

ODANA

This is rice cooked in the way you are probably used to eating it. Heat 2 cups of water to boiling. Add 1 cup of rinsed basmati rice, stir and cover. Reduce the heat to simmer and cook for 15 minutes until the rice is tender. Feel free to add 1 tablespoon of ghee, ½ teaspoon of Cumin seeds and a few spices if you like. These spices could include ginger, mint, turmeric and salt for taste.

MUNG DAHL (LENTIL SOUP)

This is a thicker soup made of mung beans, which are nourishing but gentle on the digestion. You can eat this any time as a side dish for lunch or dinner with rice or in place of rice. Here, it's a little bit thinner and can be eaten as a soup as you prepare for more complex meals. This recipe calls for asafetida (sometimes called "hing"). You can find this pungent spice at specialty grocery stores, or you can order it online. It's the spice that makes Indian food taste more authentic. You only need a pinch of this spice in any dish, but it's also an optional ingredient here.

PREPARATION TIME **30 MIN** | SERVES **2-3**

INGREDIENTS	INSTRUCTIONS
1 cup mung dal **2 cups water**	Rinse the mung dal in a mesh strainer. Heat 2 cups of water in a saucepan to boiling.
1 tsp turmeric powder **¼ tsp asafetida** **½ tsp cumin seeds** **1 green chili**	Add the mung beans, turmeric, asafetida (if using), cumin seeds, and finely chopped green chili. Cover and reduce to medium heat for 20 minutes or until it is soft. If the soup becomes too thick, you can add water as needed.
¾ tsp salt **1 tsp ginger (grated)** **3 tbsp chopped cilantro** **1 tbsp ghee / olive oil**	After cooking, you can further dilute this soup by adding 2 –2½ cups of water. Add salt and grated ginger, and cook for 5 more minutes. If you are serving this as a side dish, there is no need to dilute it after cooking.
	Before serving, garnish with cilantro and add ghee.

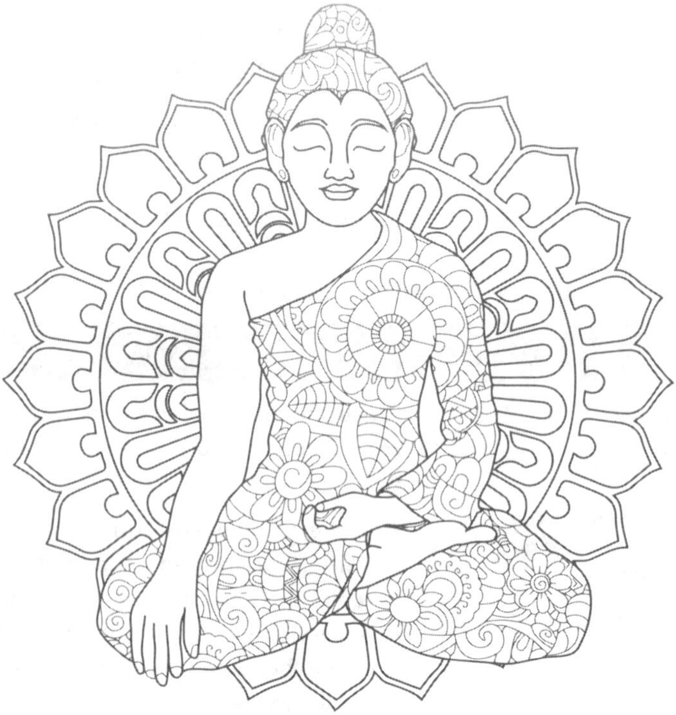

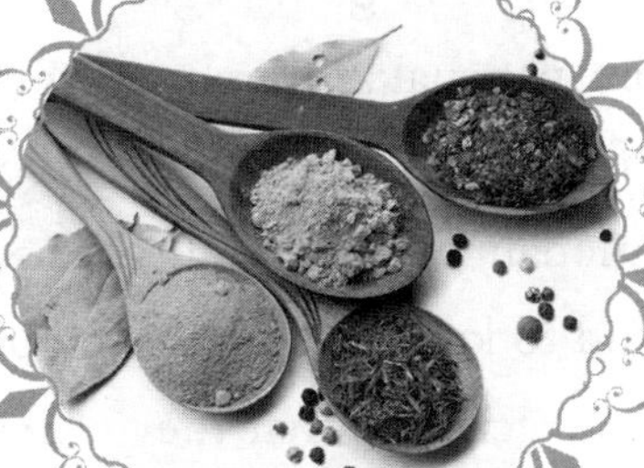

CHAPTER THIRTEEN

RECIPES FOR HEALING

The following recipes can be used any time you need a good, clean meal to get your digestive fire going again. Many people use these recipes during the pre-panchakarma phase, when they are trying to eliminate extra ama from their digestive tract before embarking on a multi-day treatment modality. They can also be used after the treatment to keep ama at bay and to keep the digestion going at full speed. The great thing about these recipes is that they are simple to prepare and very nourishing. If you are interested in adopting an Ayurvedic lifestyle of clean eating and abundant health, these recipes will be a lifeline for you. The first step is to stop by the supermarket or local health food store and pick up fresh spices that you can use in all of these recipes.

Seven Important Spices

Many of the following recipes use combinations of certain essential spices. This is no accident. These spices promote healing and vitality above all others. It's important to familiarize yourself with the ways in which these spices benefit the digestion and the body as a whole.

CUMIN

You may be familiar with cumin as a staple of Mexican cuisine when mixed with chili powder, but it's also a standby for many Ayurvedic recipes. It serves as a stimulant to the digestion, while also soothing the digestive tract. It even prevents flatulence and diarrhea while calming the stomach. While you can buy cumin powder almost anywhere, you will also want to stock up on cumin seeds for many of these recipes. This herb increases vata and pitta doshas while suppressing kapha.

CORIANDER

This is both an herb and a spice. The stalks and leaves of the coriander plant are known as cilantro, and several of these recipes use cilantro leaves. The seeds of the plant are packed with nutritive and healing value. The seeds are both stimulating to the digestion and soothing for the stomach and intestines. Ground coriander helps alleviate headaches and swelling, particularly in the joints, and is a tonic for the nervous system as a whole. Ground coriander is an ingredient used topically as well. When made into a paste, it can cover wounds and ulcers to provide healing.

TURMERIC

This intense yellow herb has a mild taste and yet it packs a punch in terms of healing properties. Turmeric is a powerful anti-inflammatory agent that you can eat in food, put into a smoothie or take in pill form. Many people take turmeric every day to relieve joint pain and reduce the chronic inflammation that can lead to many systemic disorders. It's easy to digest, and has the ability to stimulate digestion even as it is improving circulation, skin tone and the blood itself.

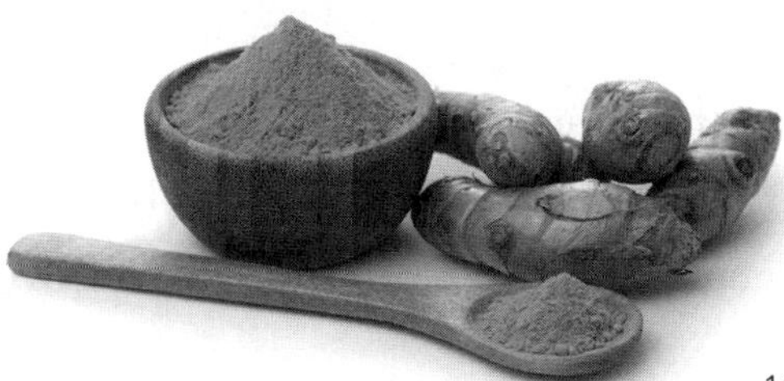

MUSTARD

This herb is known for adding mild heat to everything from salad dressings to sauces. However, its real power is its healing action. Like many spices, it stimulates the digestion, but it also sooths irritated or inflamed tissues along the digestive tract. It helps to heal bruises, relieve tooth aches, and soothe sore muscles. It can even positively affect the lungs and respiration. You will be using it in small doses where it can work in concert with other herbs. You probably have mustard powder on hand, but you should buy mustard seeds to use in most of these recipes.

ASAFETIDA

Those not familiar with Indian cooking may never have heard of this herb, which is also known as "hing." It has a pungent aroma that makes some people wary. But no Indian dish tastes authentic without a pinch of this powder. You can find it in some specialty stores and online. It will come tightly sealed and should remain so until you use it. In addition to giving Indian dishes a distinctive earthy flavor, this herb helps sooth the digestive tract, relieves pain, and stimulates the body's energy. Even in tiny doses, it is considered to be a balm for respiratory conditions, flatulence and coughing.

FENUGREEK

This is another special Indian spice that's not common, but it is very good to regulate blood sugar. It is sometimes called bitter tonic and is good for blood purification. It is also good for your bones. Lots of curry mixes contain fenugreek because it rounds out and compliments many other spices. As a health food, it helps in digestion, and slows the absorption of sugars into the blood stream, which helps regulate blood sugar levels. It also helps to reduce inflammation.

GINGER

This herb is used in everything from baking to savory dishes. You can find it powdered or you can buy the raw bulb in most supermarkets. Simply peel the outer skin and then slice or chop the meat of the bulb. This spice is pleasantly pungent. Ginger has long been known for its benefits for digestion. It cools and calms the stomach and can relieve nausea. It reduces the symptoms of any cold or cough, and has a beneficial effect on the respiratory system.

Ghee

In Ayurveda, ghee plays an important role in cooking because of its healing properties. And because it has a high smoke point, meaning that you can cook with it at high temperatures before it starts to smoke.

Ghee is nourishing, anti-aging and rejuvenating. It's good for the eyes, kidneys, and improves digestion. Most of the recipes that follow call for ghee as the cooking oil. While it's easy to purchase ghee at most supermarkets, there is no reason why you can't make it at home. It's made by cooking butter to remove all of the milk solids and water. What is left is a shelf stable oil with exceptional flavor and aroma. From an Ayurvedic perspective, ghee is sweet in taste and has a cooling potency along with a high melting point. Research shows that it helps to reduce LDL cholesterol and triglycerides, while actually raising HDL levels.

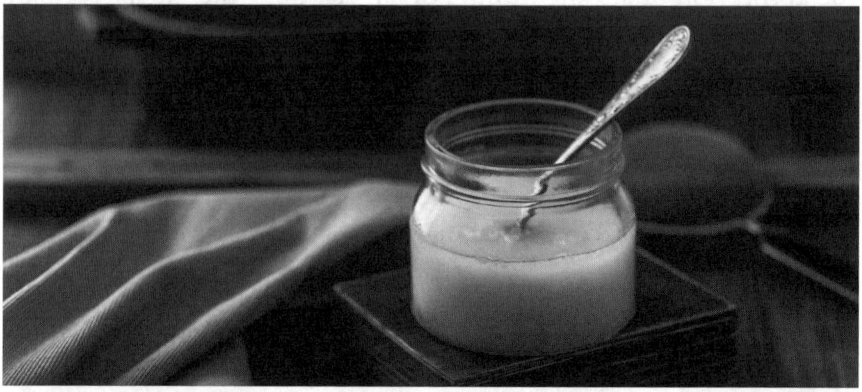

INGREDIENTS	INSTRUCTIONS
1 pound unsalted organic butter **Cheesecloth or muslin cloth or fine strainer** **Heavy-bottomed cook pot** **1 clean glass jar with lid**	Melt the butter over medium heat gradually in a heavy-bottomed pot. Do not stir. Cook the melted butter until it is a clear golden liquid. It may bubble some, and foam may form on top, but do not skim off the foam. Golden or light brown solids will form and may settle at the bottom. Butter usually begins to boil with lots of bubbles. When it is done, it will have foam on top of it, indicating that ghee is nearly done. Remove from heat while the liquid is a clear gold. A darker color means overdone ghee. When it is warm, carefully strain the ghee through the cheesecloth or with a fine strainer into a clean, dry glass jar. Close with a lid when it becomes cold. At room temperature, ghee looks semi-solid. It does not need to be refrigerated.

Chard and Mung Bean Soup

When you are ready for vegetables, this is an easy first foray into a slightly more complex meal. This contains finely chopped chard leaves that offer flavor and a little bit of fiber. This recipe requires a little bit of pre-planning because you will want to soak the beans for at least a half hour before you begin cooking. This recipe is for a soup, but you can reduce the amount of water by up to one half and make a more traditional dal to be served as a side dish for any meal. It can also be a complete meal if served over basmati rice.

PRESOAKING TIME **30 MIN** | PREPARATION TIME **10 MIN** | SERVES **2**

INGREDIENTS	INSTRUCTIONS
½ cup green split mung beans **3-4 stems of chard, finely chopped** **1 ½ tbsp olive oil** **¼ tsp cumin seeds** **⅛ tsp mustard seeds** **⅛ tsp asafetida (hing)** **½ tsp turmeric powder** **¼ tsp chili powder** **Pinch of salt** **1 tbsp fresh coconut, grated**	Soak split mung dal for at least 30 minutes in 2 cups of warm water. Wash and stem the chard, then chop the leaves finely. Heat the oil in the pan. Add the cumin and mustard seeds. Add the asafetida, turmeric and chili powder. Let the spices heat through while you stir for 30 seconds to 1 minute. Then add beans and water. Stir, cover and cook on medium low heat for 10 to 15 minutes until the beans are soft. Add the salt and chopped chard. Stir and cook uncovered for 5 more minutes. Add the grated coconut. Serve hot.

Khichadi

This traditional Ayurvedic dish is one of the most nourishing meals you will ever find. It combines the aromatic basmati rice with the cooling and grounding effect of mung dal. The spices add fuel to your digestive fire and the vegetables feed your cells without causing stress to the digestive tract. This is a go-to comfort food in India in part because it is so tasty, but also because it can be adapted in endless ways. It is also popular because anyone at any age can safely eat this soup.

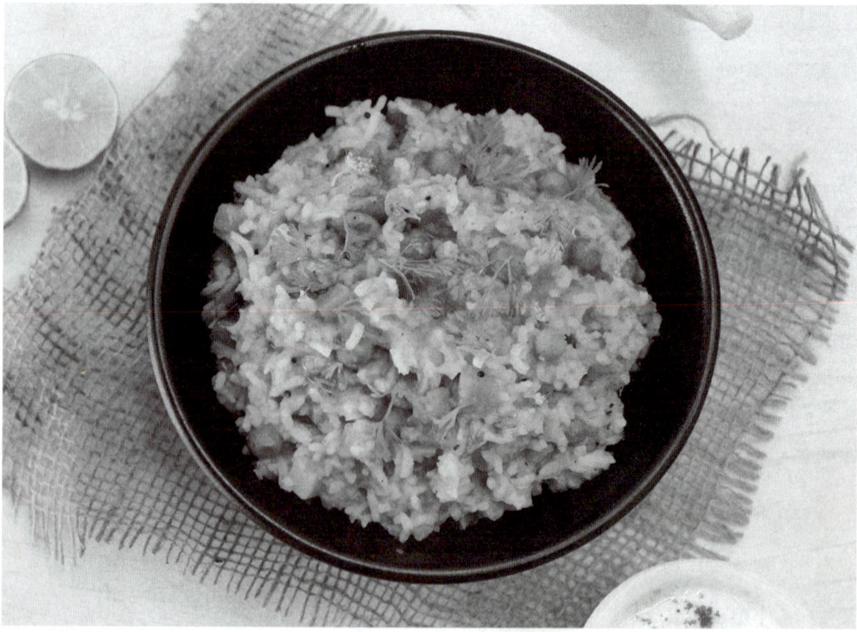

PREPARATION TIME **20 MIN** | SERVES **2-3**

INGREDIENTS	INSTRUCTIONS
½ cup organic basmati rice ¼ cup mung dal (yellow lentils) 1 tbsp ghee 1 tsp cumin seeds ½ tsp mustard seeds 1 tsp turmeric ½ tsp red chili powder or paprika powder ¼ tsp cinnamon powder 1 tsp grated ginger 1 tsp salt 4 cups of water 1 cup carrot, peeled and cut into small slices 1 cup zucchini, washed and cut into thin rounds or small pieces	Rinse the rice and beans well. Put them into a bowl with enough water to cover them and soak them for at least 30 minutes or up to two hours. Soaking the rice and beans helps them to cook faster. You can omit this step if you don't want to wait, or if you forget, but then increase the cooking time by 10 minutes. Heat ghee in the pot and add cumin seeds, mustard seeds, turmeric, chili powder, cinnamon and ginger. Sauté for two minutes on medium heat. Drain all the water from the rice and lentils and add them to the pot. Stir for 2 to 3 minutes to heat the rice and beans and to let them absorb some of the spices. Add water to the pot and bring to a boil. Then reduce the heat back to medium low and cook for 10 to 15 minutes. Add vegetables and cook uncovered for an additional 5 to 7 minutes until the vegetables have become tender. Adjust the spices to taste, adding a pinch of salt for taste and serve hot with ghee on top. This dish is very versatile. If you prefer a thicker soup, you can reduce the water by one cup. If you like a consistency that more resembles soup, you can add more than the recommended 4 cups or you can add a little water in the last step.

Tridoshic Kichadi

Once you become comfortable making khichadi, you will want to experiment and try new versions. This recipe adds green beans, cilantro and extra spices. The combination nourishes all of the doshas and is a perfect dish to try after a panchakarma, when your body is feeling its best. It's also a good recipe for any time. It can be a simple lunch, a clean and easy dinner or a side dish or soup served before a bigger meal. This meal serves several people, so it's perfect for a weeknight when you are trying to get your family to share your healthy lifestyle.

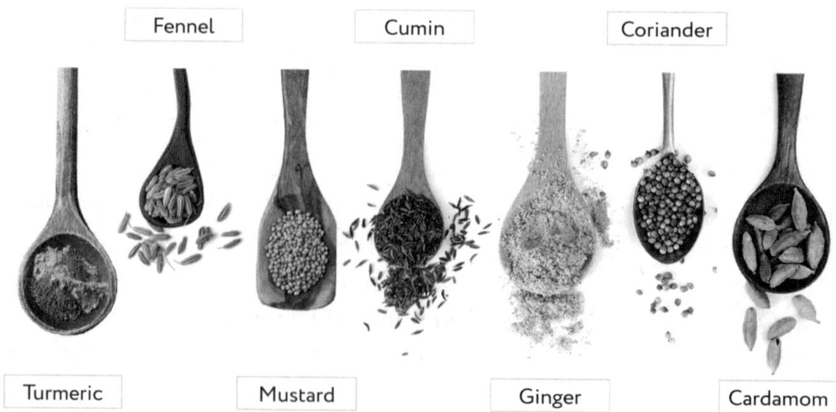

PRESOAKING TIME **5 MIN** | PREPARATION TIME **30 MIN** | SERVES **7-8**

INGREDIENTS	INSTRUCTIONS
2 cups Basmati rice	Wash rice and mung dal until water is clear. Wash green beans and chop into 1-inch pieces.
1 cup split mung dal	Warm the ghee in a sauce pan. Add turmeric, fennel, mustard seeds, cumin seeds and sauté for 1 to 2 minutes, long enough for the spices to become aromatic, but not to brown.
2 cups French green beans	Add rice and mung and sauté for another couple of minutes to allow them to absorb the spices.
2 tbsp ghee	Add ginger and green beans, stir sauté for 1 more minute.
½ tsp turmeric	Add 6 to 6 ½ cups of water and bring to a boil.
1 tsp fennel seeds	After Kichadi has come to a boil, add salt and reduce to medium low heat. Cover and cook until tender for 30 to 45 minutes, adding water as needed to keep the mixture moist or to make it soupy, if that is your preference.
1 tsp mustard seeds	Before serving, add the coriander powder and stir well. Garnish with powdered cardamom and fresh chopped cilantro.
1 ½ tsp cumin seeds	
1 tbsp grated ginger	
2 tsp salt	
1 tbsp coriander powder	
4 pods of cardamom (peeled and ground) or 1 tsp powdered	
1 bunch of finely chopped cilantro	

Mixed Vegetables

If you need a quick and easy evening meal, this is the perfect recipe. It comes together with a little bit of prep time chopping vegetables and cooks in just ten minutes.

PREPARATION TIME **10 MIN** | SERVES **1-2**

INGREDIENTS

5 to 6 stalks of asparagus

1 zucchini

1 cup cabbage, chopped

½ cumin seeds

½ tsp turmeric powder

¼ tsp asafetida (hing) powder

Salt to taste

Black pepper to taste

2 tbsp coconut oil or ghee

INSTRUCTIONS

Wash the asparagus, cabbage and zucchini thoroughly.

Cut asparagus in small pieces and cut zucchini into 1" thin and 3" long slices. Chop the cabbage.

Over medium heat, add oil to a skillet large enough to accommodate the vegetables. Add cumin seeds, hing and turmeric along with the vegetables.

Stir the vegetables, then cover the skillet and let it cook for 8 to 10 minutes.

Stir it properly and serve hot.

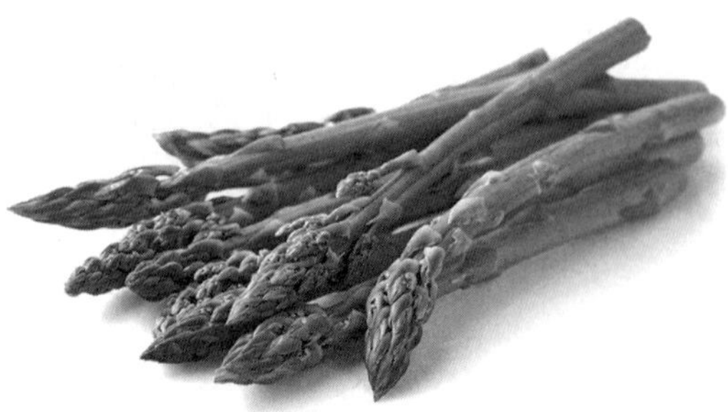

Bok Choy Broccoli

This is another easy vegetable recipe that you can eat as a meal on its own, or you can serve it as a side dish for any meal. The flavors of broccoli and bok choy come alive with the ghee and lemon juice that make for a nice, light vinaigrette.

PREPARATION TIME **10 MIN** | SERVES **2-3**

INGREDIENTS

- 2 tbsp ghee
- 1 medium onion, thinly sliced
- 1 tbsp fresh ginger root, grated or minced
- 2 cloves garlic, crushed
- ½ tsp salt
- 3 cups fresh broccoli florets, sliced
- 1 pound bok choy, coarsely chopped
- 2 tsp lemon juice

INSTRUCTIONS

Heat the oil in a skillet on medium high heat. Add onion, ginger, garlic, and salt.

Sauté 2 to 3 minutes until the spices become golden and aromatic.

Add the broccoli and bok choy and stir-fry for 5 to 7 more minutes.

Squeeze lemon juice on top before serving.

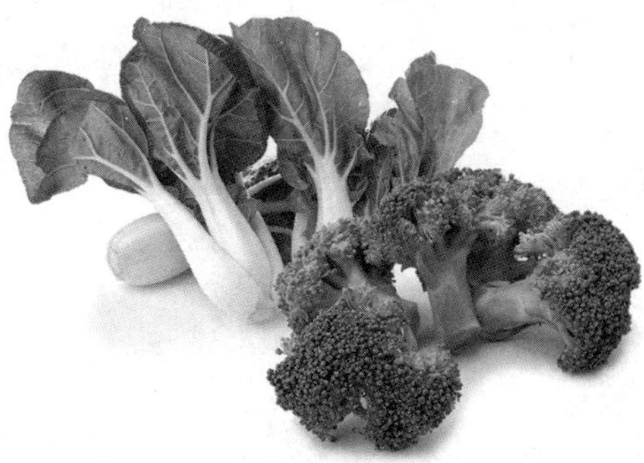

HEALTHY SOUPS

Nothing is more nourishing or grounding than a vegetable soup. These are complete meals on their own. They contain plenty of fiber and dense nutrients that will fill you up while leaving you feeling light and refreshed.

Ayurvedic Vegetable Soup

This unique blend of herbs and vegetables means that this soup balances all of the doshas. The unusual mix of cabbage, sweet carrots and yams makes this soup ideal for fall, winter and spring. It's particularly healthy to eat this soup at the fall and spring equinox, and in mid-December when the doshas are on the move and may need a little help rebalancing for the new season.

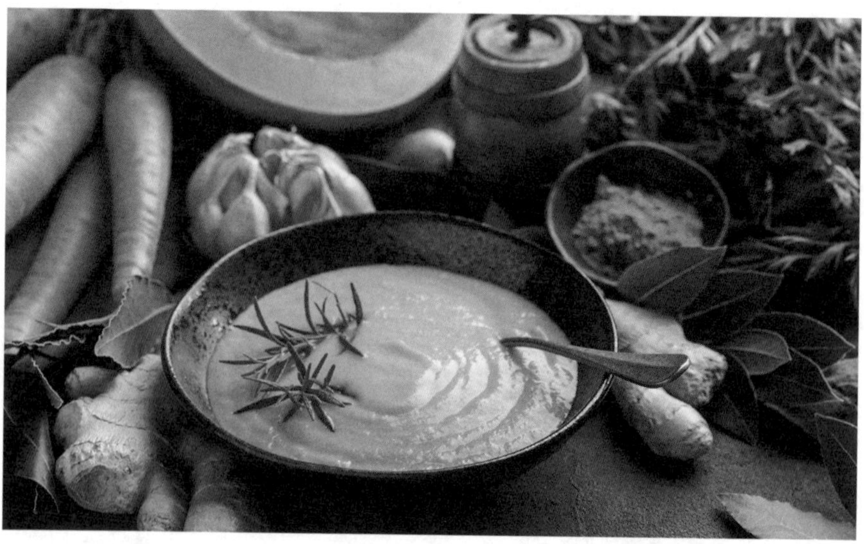

PREPARATION TIME **20 MIN** | SERVES **3-4**

INGREDIENTS	INSTRUCTIONS
1 big onion, chopped **½ cabbage, sliced finely and chopped** **1 medium carrot, chopped** **1 small yam, chopped** **1 tbsp olive oil** **5 cups water** **1 ½ tsp grated ginger** **1 ½ tsp coriander powder** **¼ tsp cayenne** **½ tsp cumin powder** **½ tsp turmeric powder** **1 tsp salt** **1 tbsp lemon juice**	Wash all the vegetables and chop finely. Heat the oil in a big soup pot. Add the onion and sauté for 3 minutes. Add the other vegetables and sauté for 2 minutes. Add 2 cups of water, ginger, turmeric, cayenne, and salt and cook for 10 minutes. Add coriander and cumin powder and cook for 15 more minutes. Add 3 cups of water and cook for 5 more minutes. Before serving, add lemon juice and mix well. Serve hot.

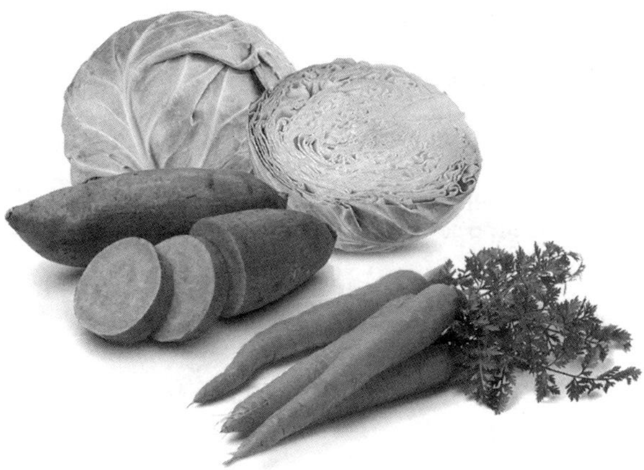

Lentil Soup

This classic soup has been updated to fit the Ayurvedic lifestyle. It contains plenty of vegetables and traditional spices that promote healing and vibrant digestion.

PREPARATION TIME **30-45 MIN** | SERVES **6-7**

INGREDIENTS

- 1 cup French lentils
- 4 cups water
- 1 medium onion
- 1 clove garlic
- 1 medium carrot
- 1 tbsp ghee
- 1 tsp coriander powder
- 1 tsp cumin seeds
- ½ tsp cayenne powder
- ½ tsp cumin powder
- ½ cup spinach leaves, chopped
- Pinch of sea salt

INSTRUCTIONS

Rinse the lentils and look over them to pick out any stones or debris.

Wash and cut all vegetables into small pieces.

Heat the oil in a soup pot. Add cumin seeds and onion and sauté till the onion softens and turns golden.

Add lentils, carrots and 2 cups of water. Cover and cook for 10 minutes.

Add cumin, coriander, ginger, cayenne and salt, cook for 10 more minutes or until lentils are completely cooked.

Add finely chopped spinach and cook for 5 minutes.

Dilute by adding 2 cups of water.

Serve hot.

Spinach Broccoli Soup

This simple soup comes together in a few minutes. You sauté the vegetables, then puree them into a smooth soup with just a light touch of spices to round out the flavors. It is densely packed with nutrients and perfect for any busy work night.

PREPARATION TIME **10 MIN** | SERVES **2-3**

INGREDIENTS	INSTRUCTIONS
1 tbsp ghee or olive oil	In a large pan, heat the ghee, then sauté onion, and garlic till it turns golden.
¼ cup onion, finely chopped	Add the chopped spinach and broccoli and sauté on medium heat for 4 to 5 minutes until they are cooked.
1 clove garlic, finely chopped	Remove from heat and let it cool for a few minutes.
4-5 cups spinach leaves, chopped	Transfer the vegetables to a blender and puree until smooth.
2 cups broccoli pieces	Add water as needed to make the puree the consistency of soup.
3-4 cups water	Return the puree to the soup pot and heat to boiling.
½ tsp pepper, crushed	Add the pepper and cumin and salt to taste.
½ tsp cumin powder	Serve hot and garnish with additional ghee.
Salt to taste	

Celery Broccoli Soup

This is a smooth, creamy soup without the cream. Both the celery and broccoli are pureed and accented with the Six Taste Spice Mix that's available from Ayurvedic Healing. You can also mix your own spices, including cumin, coriander, turmeric, ground fennel, cinnamon, salt, ground fenugreek, ginger and cayenne. (But it's easier to buy the spice mix, which can be used in any dish).

PREPARATION TIME **10 MIN** | SERVES **2-3**

INGREDIENTS	INSTRUCTIONS
2 stalks of celery **1 tbsp olive oil or ghee** **6 cups water or vegetable broth** **2 cups broccoli** **Salt to taste** **Six Taste Spice Mix to taste**	Steam the broccoli and celery until medium soft. Blend together with the water or vegetable broth in a blender until smooth. Pour the pureed vegetables into a pot and add salt, oil and Six Taste Spice Mix. Stir and serve hot.

KHICHADI VARIATIONS

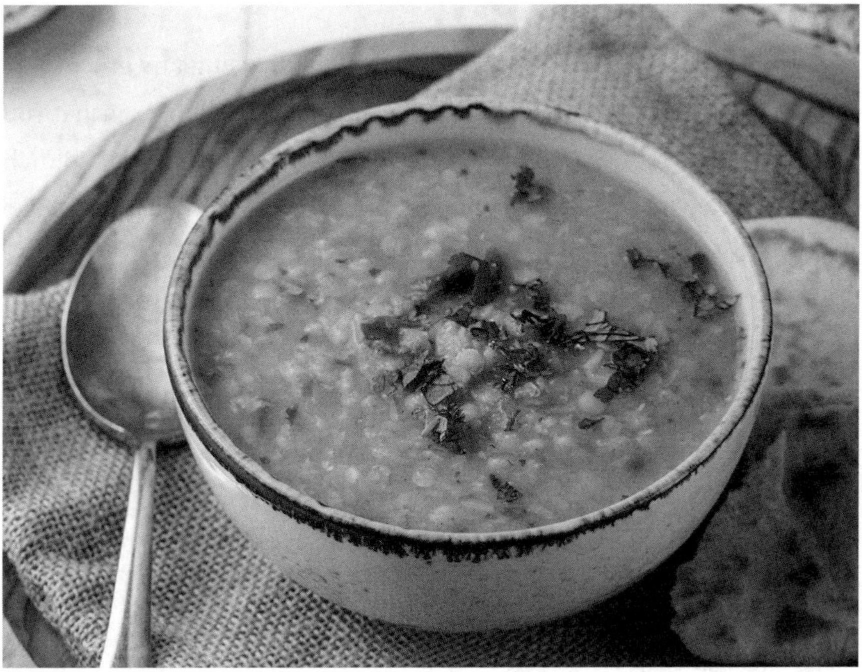

One of the best things about this traditional dish is that it can be adapted to nearly endless variations. The following recipes show how to use different vegetables, grains and spices to adapt to every season and every mood. This will be the dish that you turn to every time your body needs a clean and easily prepared meal.

Khichadi with Baby Carrots and Greens

This is the most basic variation on khichadi, using any greens you have in the fridge, or any greens you see at the farmer's market that you want to chop and use. This could be something as simple as a bunch of spinach leaves, or kale, swiss chard, or even dandelion leaves. It also features carrots that add fiber and sweetness to the dish.

PREPARATION TIME **20-25 MIN** | SERVES **2-3**

INGREDIENTS	INSTRUCTIONS
½ cup of organic split green mung beans	Warm ghee or oil in a pot.
1 cup of white organic basmati rice	Add mustard seeds, cumin, coriander, turmeric, ginger and sauté for just a few minutes to let them become aromatic but not to brown.
1 tbsp of ghee /coconut oil	Add the beans and rice and stir to let the spices mix with the grains.
1 tsp of cumin seeds	Add 4 to 5 cups of water, and bring to a boil.
½ tsp of cumin powder	Add salt, cover and reduce heat to low.
1 tsp coriander powder	Cook for 35 - 40 minutes until the beans and rice are very soft.
½ tsp mustard seeds	Add veggies and cook another 10 to 15 minutes. This will produce a thick stew.
¼-½ tsp cayenne pepper (optional)	Feel free to add more water depending on what consistency you like.
½ tsp salt	
1 tsp ginger (fresh, grated)	
½ cup baby carrots	
1 cup dark leafy greens washed and chopped.	

Khichadi with Buckwheat

Buckwheat has an earthy, nutty flavor that's tempered by the green mung beans in this soup. Despite the name, this grain is not wheat related, and contains no gluten. It does contain both protein and fiber along with many antioxidants. You can serve this as a side dish to steamed vegetables or salads or it is a complete meal on its own.

PREPARATION TIME **20 MIN** | SERVES **2-3**

INGREDIENTS	INSTRUCTIONS
5 cups water	Bring the water to a boil in a large stainless steel pot.
1 cup buckwheat	Wash the buckwheat and mung beans, and add to boiling water. Add salt.
½ cup slit green mung beans	Cover and simmer on low heat for 20 minutes.
¼ tsp Himalayan salt	In a small cast iron skillet, heat the ghee or oil and add the cumin seeds.
1 tsp ghee or olive oil	When the seeds turn golden brown, pour the mixture into the khichadi.
1 tsp cumin seeds	Stir, cover and continue to simmer for an additional five minutes over low heat.
	Serve warm.

Millet Khichadi

Millet is one of the easiest grains to digest and one of the least allergenic, so it's safe for everyone to eat. It has a nutty flavor that's a bit like quinoa. It's rich in protein, fiber and B vitamins, iron, calcium and magnesium. It's a favorite grain for those who are trying to lose weight because it's so filling and densely nutritious.

PREPARATION TIME **40 MIN** | SERVES **2**

INGREDIENTS	INSTRUCTIONS
½ cup millet **3-4 cups water** **½ cup split green mung beans** **¼ tsp Himalayan salt** **1 cup baby spinach** **1 tsp olive oil/ghee** **1 tsp cumin seeds** **½ tsp turmeric powder**	Bring the water to a boil in a large stainless steel pot. Wash the millet and mung beans and add to boiling water. Add salt. Cover and simmer on low heat for 20 minutes. In a small cast iron skillet, heat the ghee or oil and add the cumin seeds, turmeric. Sauté the seeds until they turn golden brown, then pour the mixture into the khichari. Stir, cover and add baby spinach and continue to simmer for an additional 5 to 7 minutes over low heat. Serve warm.

Quinoa Khichadi

Quinoa is all the rage because it's a nutty, crunchy alternative to rice. It's gluten free and full of protein and fiber along with all nine essential amino acids. This ancient grain is considered one of the best sources of plant protein available. When mixed with mung beans and seeds and spices, it becomes a nearly perfect one dish meal.

PREPARATION TIME **20 MIN** | SERVES **2**

INGREDIENTS	INSTRUCTIONS
1 cup organic quinoa	Wash and Drain quinoa and lentils and add to the cooking pot along with the water.
½ cup organic yellow mung beans	Bring to a boil, and add the curry powder.
1 tsp curry powder	Boil uncovered over medium heat, stirring occasionally for 15 to 20 minutes.
4-5 stems of cilantro, with leaves	It's nearly done when you dip a stirring ladle in and find no water at the bottom of the pot. Make sure to remove the pot from heat if the quinoa seems to be sticking to the pot.
1 tsp sesame seeds, 1 tsp sunflower seeds, and 1 tsp chia seeds	Turn off the heat and add all seeds. Stir well, and cover.
2-3 tsp olive oil	Let it sit covered for five minutes while the last of the water gets absorbed.
3 cups of water	Garnish with finely chopped cilantro and serve hot.

Quinoa and Amaranth Khichadi

Amaranth has a fine texture similar to cous cous and as a result, some home cooks find it an intimidating ingredient to work with. In this recipe, we combine it with the more familiar quinoa, so that the slightly sweet and delicate amaranth gets backed up by the crunch and taste of quinoa. Add a few vegetables and a few nuts and this makes a nice, easy lunch or dinner recipe.

PREPARATION TIME **20 MIN** | SERVES **2**

INGREDIENTS	INSTRUCTIONS
½ cup organic quinoa	Rinse the quinoa and amaranth thoroughly through a fine mesh strainer. It does not have to dry completely.
2 tbsp organic amaranth	Heat up the oil and add mustard seed, cumin seed & cayenne pepper.
Salt to taste	Add 1 ½ cups of water and let it come to a boil.
1-2 tbsp oil or ghee	Add salt, quinoa, amaranth and cook till the water is absorbed.
½ tsp cumin seeds	Add finely chopped spinach, cilantro and baby carrots while the quinoa is cooking on the stove top.
¼ tsp cayenne pepper or black pepper powder	Fluff it up, add nuts and seeds and a little bit of ghee on top before serving.
¼ tsp mustard seeds	
5-6 baby carrots	
¼ cup spinach or Swiss chard, finely chopped	
4-5 stems cilantro with leaves	
5-6 walnuts or almonds, chopped	
2 tsp seeds, either sesame, sunflower or pumpkin	

Khichadi with Brown Basmati Rice and Sprouted Mung Beans

This recipe calls for brown basmati rice, which has a deeper nutty flavor and more fiber than the white rice. It also teaches you how to make mung bean sprouts. You won't be using the split mung beans as in dal recipes. Instead, you'll use whole mung beans and soak them overnight so that they can sprout a little bit, which makes them more nutritious.

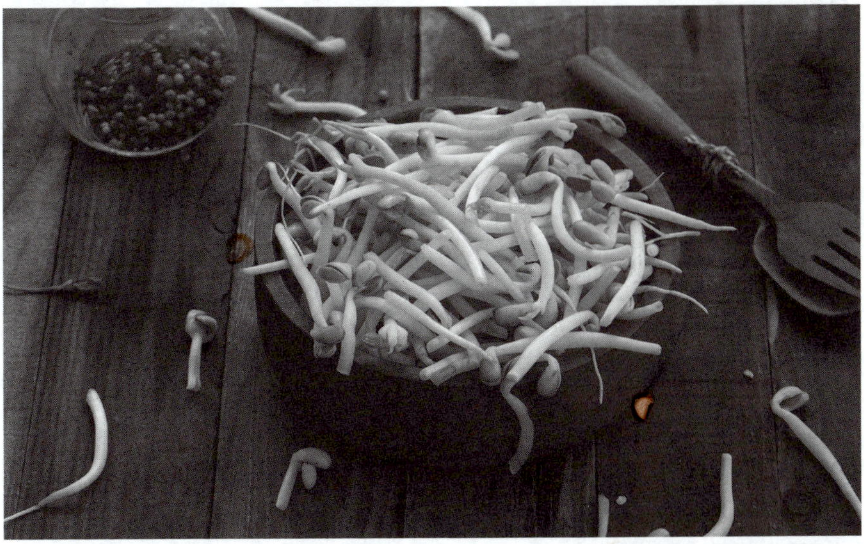

PREPARATION TIME **25-30 MIN** | SERVES **2-3**

INGREDIENTS	INSTRUCTIONS
½ cup organic whole green mung beans **½ cup organic brown basmati rice** **½ tsp dry roasted coriander seeds powder** **½ tsp dry roasted cumin seeds powder** **3-4 tsp ghee** **1 tsp garlic, finely chopped** **½ tsp turmeric powder** **½ tsp fresh ground black pepper** **½ cup chopped or grated carrots** **½ cup chopped parsnips** **½ cup mixture of chopped spinach, basil and green onion** **1 tsp chopped fresh ginger** **½ tsp pink Himalayan salt** **Juice of ½ lime or lemon**	Soak the rice and beans overnight in water. In the morning, drain the water and rinse the rice and beans in a fine mesh strainer. Combine these together with the chopped carrot and parsnip and cook in the rice cooker. If you don't have a rice cooker, put the rice, beans and veggies in a saucepan with 1 cup of water. Bring the water to a boil and then cover and reduce the heat to low. Simmer for 20 minutes or until the grains are tender. Put the coriander and cumin seeds in a dry skillet and roast on medium heat until aromatic and slightly browned. Then grind them to powder in a spice grinder or use a mortar and pestle. Heat the ghee in a second pan and add the garlic, sautéing it until it is golden-brown. Add cumin, coriander and other spices to taste. Add finely chopped spinach, basil and green onion and sauté briefly. Combine everything together into the rice cooker. Add the salt and lime juice. Stir and enjoy.

TEAS AND OTHER HEALTHY DRINKS

Once you adopt a healthy Ayurvedic lifestyle, you will want the kinds of teas and other beverages that can help keep your doshas balanced and healthy. Use these recipes to alleviate symptoms and preserve your energy throughout the year.

Kanji

The first few days after your panchakarma treatment, you will not have much of an appetite. You will need to stoke the digestive fire in order to revive your energy. This healthy rice-based drink is useful to sip on those days when you want a little nutrition but don't feel like eating. This drink is also handy whenever you fast. Make a batch of this in the morning, put the liquid into a thermos and sip throughout the day.

PREPARATION TIME **20 MIN**

INGREDIENTS	INSTRUCTIONS
7 parts water **1 part organic brown rice, pinch of salt, fresh ground ginger, and cumin**	Bring water and rice to a boil and continue to cook uncovered until the rice becomes swollen and broken. Stir and strain out the rice. However, it is not necessary to strain out small pieces of rice. Add a pinch each of ginger, ground cumin and salt. Pour into a thermos and drink throughout the day.

Morning Smoothie

This smoothie is the basis for endless variations. It offers a quick breakfast that you can enjoy at home or on the go. Use whatever berries you have. You can substitute many kinds of greens for the spinach. Add ¼ avocado if you like, or soak ¼ cup of nuts overnight and add those to the mix.

PREPARATION TIME **5 MIN** | SERVES **1**

INGREDIENTS	INSTRUCTIONS
1 cup liquid (water, coconut water, or rice milk) **1 scoop pea, hemp, or rice protein powder** **1 tbsp flax seed, chia seed, or hemp seed** **½ - 1 cup berries (raspberry, blueberry, or strawberry)** **¼ - 1 cup spinach, kale, or other leafy green** **1 tbsp coconut or flaxseed oil**	Combine all ingredients in a blender and puree until smooth. Serve immediately.

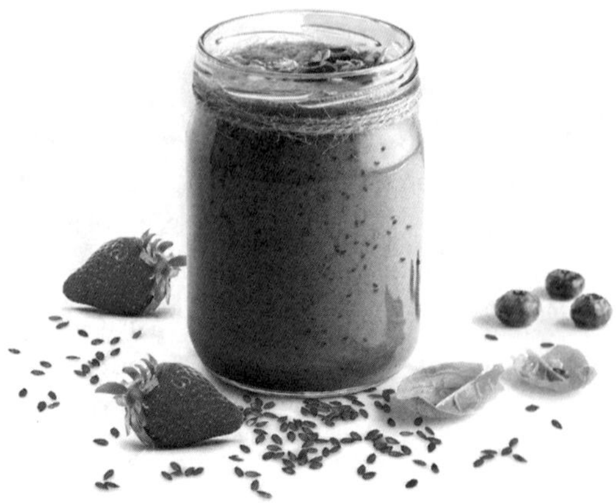

Tasty Ginger Mixture

This simple mixture contains all of the six tastes and it helps curb food cravings if you take a small amount of this before any meal. Mix this drink and keep it covered in the fridge and drink just ¼ teaspoon of this before each meal. You will find yourself eating less while feeling satisfied. In this way it helps to promote healthy eating.

PREPARATION TIME **5 MIN**

INGREDIENTS	INSTRUCTIONS
2 tsp freshly grated ginger **4-5 tsp honey or Sucanat or date sugar** **¼ tsp Himalayan salt** **¼ tsp black pepper** **2 tsp lemon juice**	Combine all these ingredients in a glass container and keep refrigerated. Before meals, take a ¼ teaspoon of the mixture and place it on your tongue. This will improve Agni, stimulate appetite and aid in digestion. The mixture will last up to a month (refrigerated).

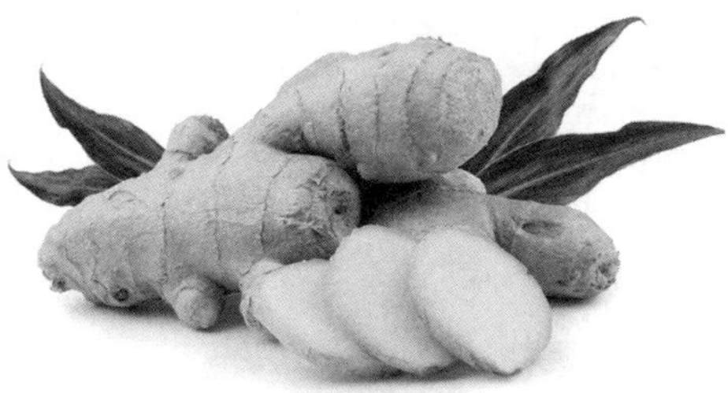

Kapha Balancing Tea

This tea helps the body prepare for the spring season. It's best to drink this tea between February and June when kapha is dominant. The warming spices promote cleansing, aid digestion and stimulate the digestion. They help flush extra fluids from the body and help keep seasonal colds at bay.

PREPARATION TIME **5 MIN** | SERVES **1**

INGREDIENTS	INSTRUCTIONS
4 cups water	In a medium saucepan, boil the water, then add the spices.
½ tsp cinnamon or crushed cinnamon sticks	Boil for 2 minutes.
½ tsp turmeric	Strain and serve.
1 tsp fennel seeds	
1 tsp grated ginger	
¼ tsp black pepper	

Pitta Balancing Tea

Drink this tea between June and the end of October to help your body deal with the high heat of summer and the increase in your daily activity. The herbs in this tea help to cool the body. The herbs in this tea help to reduce inflammation, which is more problematic during the summer months.

PREPARATION TIME **5 MIN** | SERVES **1**

INGREDIENTS	INSTRUCTIONS
4 cups water	In a medium saucepan, boil the water, then add the mint leaves and fennel.
1 tbsp crushed or chopped mint leaves	Let it steep for 3 to 4 minutes.
1 tsp fennel seeds	Remove the saucepan from the heat and let cool before straining.
2 tsp lemon juice	Then add lemon juice.
	Serve warm or cool, but don't add ice.

Vata Balancing Tea

Prepare this tea between October and the end of February when the weather is cold and dry. The herbs in this tea will keep you warm and hydrated during the winter months. This tea will help regulate your appetite and your digestion, which can become variable during the cold season.

PREPARATION TIME **5 MIN** | SERVES **1**

INGREDIENTS	INSTRUCTIONS
4 cups water	Boil the water in a saucepan.
2 tsp cumin seeds	Add the spices to the water.
1 tsp fennel seeds	Boil for 3 to 4 minutes.
1 tsp freshly grated ginger	Strain and serve hot.
¼ tsp black pepper	

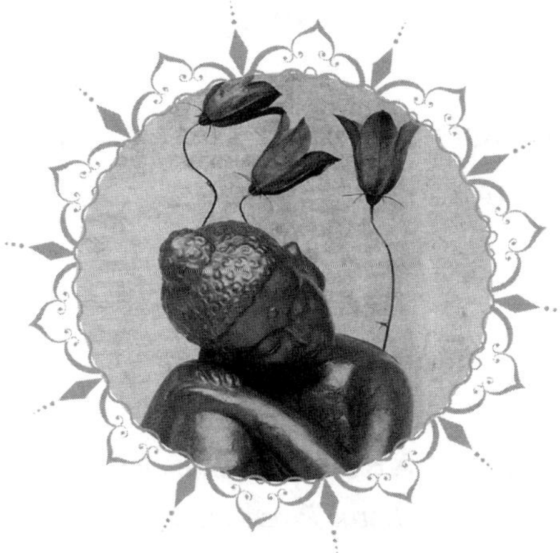

APPENDIX

Bibliography

RELEVANT BOOKS, AUDIO TITLES AND COURSES BY DR. SUHAS AND DR. MANISHA KSHIRSAGAR

The Hot Belly Diet
Simon & Schuster, 2014

Ayurveda: A quick reference handbook
Lotus Press, 2011

Enchanting Beauty:
Ancient Secrets for Inner, Outer & Lasting Beauty
Lotus Press, 2015

The Art & Science of Vedic Counseling
by David Frawley & Suhas Kshirsagar
Lotus Press, 2016

Change Your Schedule, Change Your Life
Harper Collins Publishers, 2018

Ayurvedic Wellness: The Art & Science of Vibrant Health
Audible & Audio CD set - Sounds True 2014

Effortless Weight Loss: The Ayurvedic Way
Audible & Audio CD - Sounds True 2014